LOW CARB

HIGH PROTEIN

COOKBOOK

WITH PICTURES

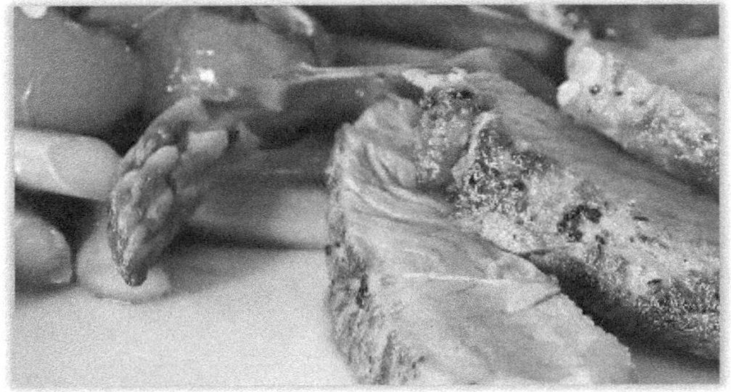

Effortless Cooking Recipes for Health, Fitness and Delicious Living.

Greg T. Oakes

TABLE OF CONTENTS

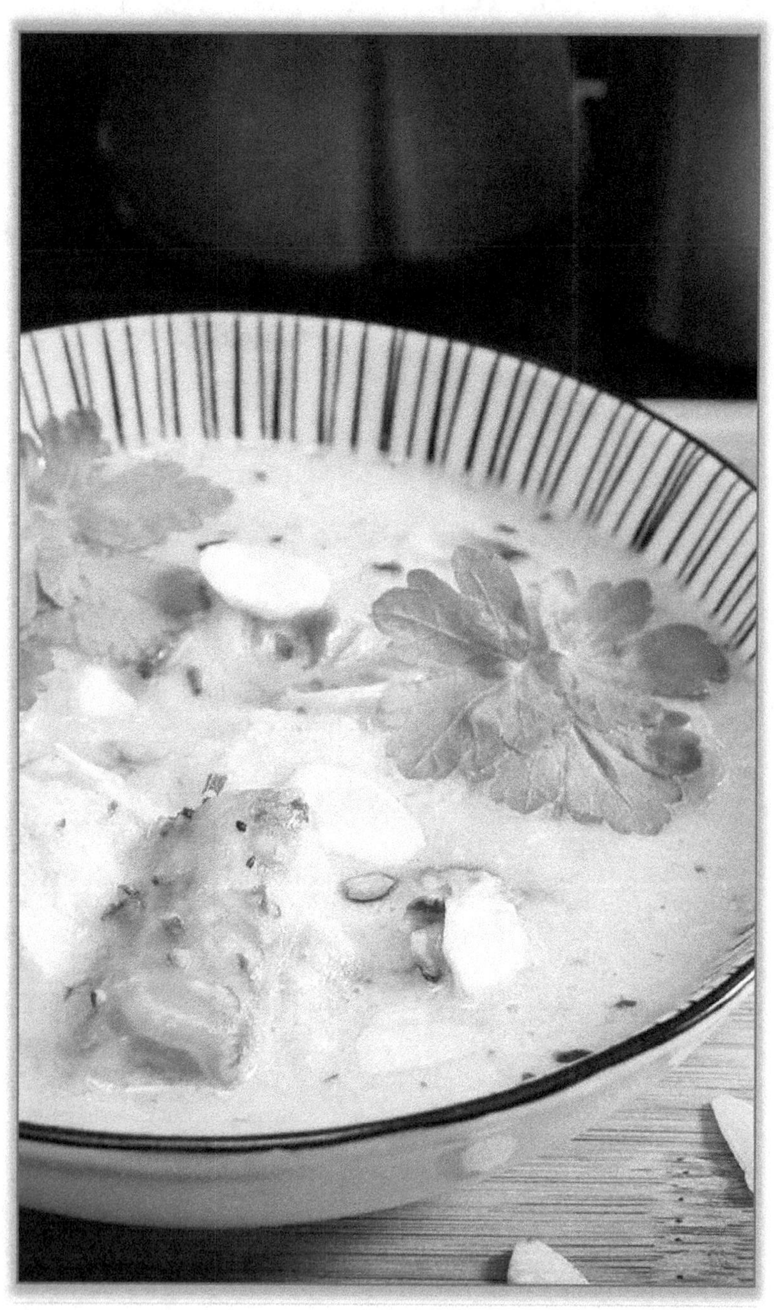

CHAPTER ONE

INTRODUCTION

A Journey to a Healthier, Happier You:

Imagine waking up feeling energized and ready to tackle the day. Imagine shedding unnecessary weight and fitting back into your favorite clothes. Imagine experiencing a newfound focus and clarity, fueled by the power of delicious and nutritious food.

This is not just a fantasy; it's a reality you can achieve with the low-carb high-protein lifestyle. This book is your guide to unlocking this transformative journey.

Have you ever felt lost in a sea of conflicting dietary advice? You're not alone. The world is bombarded with fad diets and conflicting information, leaving many people feeling confused and unsure where to turn.

But what if there was a way to eat that was not only delicious but also fueled your body with the energy it craves and helped you reach your health goals?

That's where the low-carb high-protein approach comes in. This evidence-based lifestyle has helped countless people around the world achieve incredible results, including:

- **Weight loss and improved body composition**
- **Increased energy and focus**
- **Reduced cravings and improved blood sugar control**
- **Enhanced mood and overall well-being**

This book will help you discover a world of delicious and diverse recipes that are anything but boring. From mouthwatering breakfast dishes and satisfying lunches to quick and easy snacks and hearty dinners, you'll find everything you need to embark on a culinary adventure that nourishes your body and delights your taste buds.

More than just a recipe book, this comprehensive guide will equip you with the knowledge and tools you need to succeed on your low-carb high-protein journey.

You'll learn:

- **How low-carb high-protein eating works.**
- **Essential pantry staples and cooking techniques for success.**
- **Practical tips and strategies for meal planning and prepping.**
- **Mouth-watering recipes that meets your individual needs and preferences.**
- **Answers to frequently asked questions about the diet and More!**

Throughout this journey, you'll be supported by:

- **Stunning visuals that will inspire you in the kitchen.**
- **Clear and concise instructions that are easy to follow.**

Are you ready to unlock your full potential and experience the incredible benefits of low-carb high-protein eating? **Let's begin!**

What is Low-Carb High-Protein Eating

The Low-Carb High-Protein (LCHP) diet is a nutritional strategy that emphasizes the reduction of carbohydrates while increasing the intake of protein-rich foods. The goal is to achieve a balance that promotes numerous health benefits, including weight management, improved metabolic function, and enhanced overall well-being. **Low-carb high-protein eating is like choosing a fuel-efficient car with a powerful engine.**

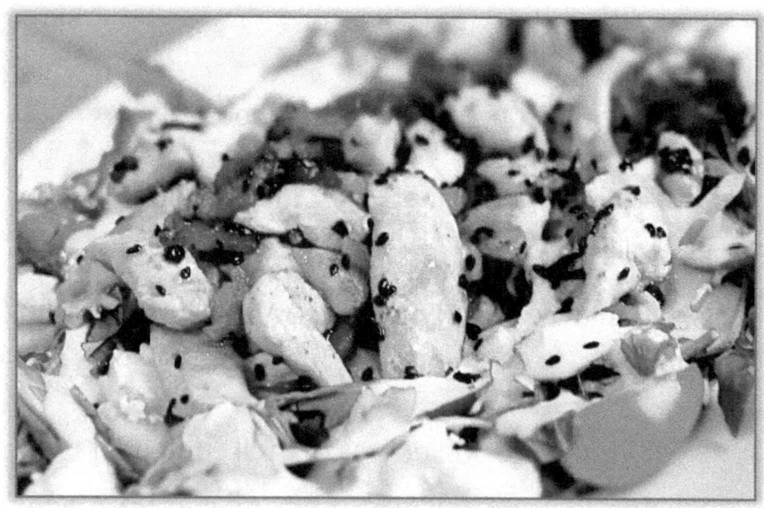

The Tremendous Benefits

1. **Improved Blood Sugar Control**
   Low-carb diets help regulate blood sugar levels, reducing the risk of type 2 diabetes and promoting weight management.

2. **Increased Energy and Focus**
   Protein provides sustained energy, allowing you to feel energized throughout the day and focus on your tasks.

3. **Reduced Cravings**
   Protein keeps you feeling full and satisfied, reducing cravings for unhealthy snacks and sugary treats.

4. **Enhanced Weight Loss**
   By burning more stored fat for energy, the low-carb high-protein approach can aid in weight loss and promote a healthy body composition.

5. **Overall Well-being**
   This dietary approach promotes various health benefits, including improved mood, better sleep, and increased physical performance.

Start Low-Carb, High-Protein Journey

Here are some practical tips to make your transition smooth and enjoyable:

1. **Start Small**
    Like a dimmer switch, begin by gradually reducing your carb intake and increasing your protein consumption. This allows your body time to adjust and minimizes any potential discomfort.

2. **Embrace Protein Power**
    Choose lean meats, fish, eggs, dairy products, legumes, and protein powders to ensure your body receives the fuel it needs for optimal health and performance.

3. **Befriend Low-Carb Veggies**
    Add essential vitamins, minerals, fiber, and flavor to your meals with options like leafy greens, broccoli, cauliflower, peppers, and mushrooms to

4. **Stock Your Kitchen**

Having the right ingredients on hand makes healthy eating easier and more convenient. Stock your pantry with low-carb staples like nuts, seeds, nut butters, healthy oils, and spices.

5. **Plan and Prep**
   Planning your meals and prepping ingredients in advance takes the stress out of healthy eating. Cook in bulk, portion out meals, and store them in the refrigerator or freezer for easy grab-and-go options.

6. **Embrace Hydration**
   Water is essential for optimal health, and it's crucial when transitioning to a low-carb diet. Aim to drink plenty of water throughout the day to stay hydrated, support digestion, and manage cravings.

7. **Be Kind to Yourself**
   Transitioning to a new diet takes time and effort. Don't be discouraged by occasional setbacks.

With these practical tips and the guidance within this book, you'll be well-equipped to embark on a successful low-carb high-protein journey.

Remember, the key is to be patient, consistent, and kind to yourself. So, take a deep breath, grab your apron, and let's start cooking your way to a healthier, happier you!

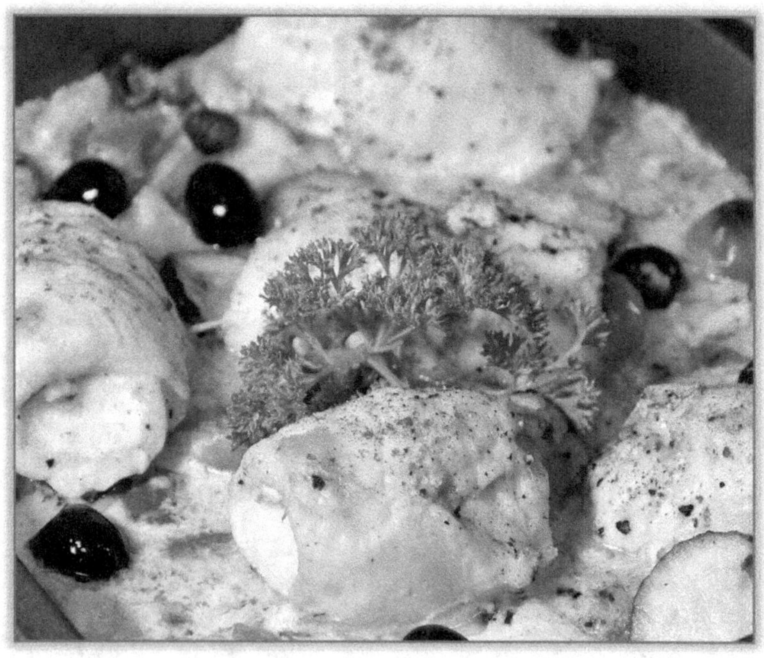

FOUNDATIONAL KNOWLEDGE

Essential Pantry Staples

Stocking your pantry with the right ingredients is crucial for success on a low-carb high-protein diet. These staples provide the foundation for countless delicious and nutritious meals, making healthy eating convenient and enjoyable.

Here are some essential pantry staples you should always have on hand:

PROTEIN POWERHOUSES

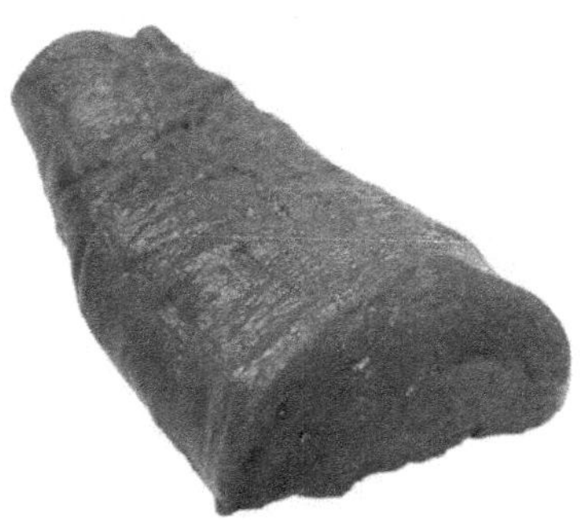

Lean meats: Chicken breast, turkey breast, lean ground beef, pork tenderloin, fish (salmon, tuna, tilapia)

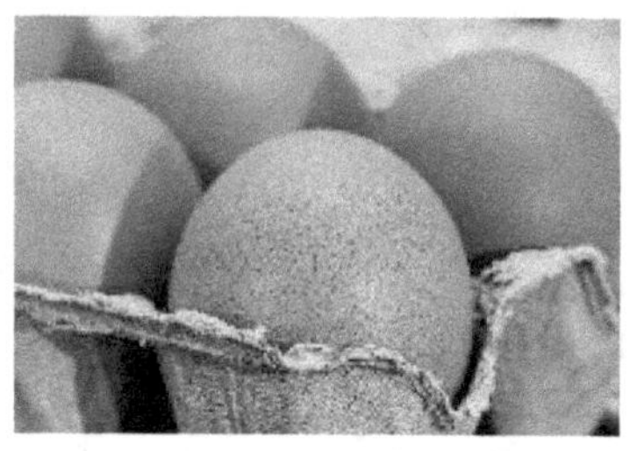

Eggs:
A versatile and affordable source of protein, perfect for breakfast, lunch, or dinner.

Legumes:
Beans, lentils, chickpeas offer protein, fiber, and essential nutrients.

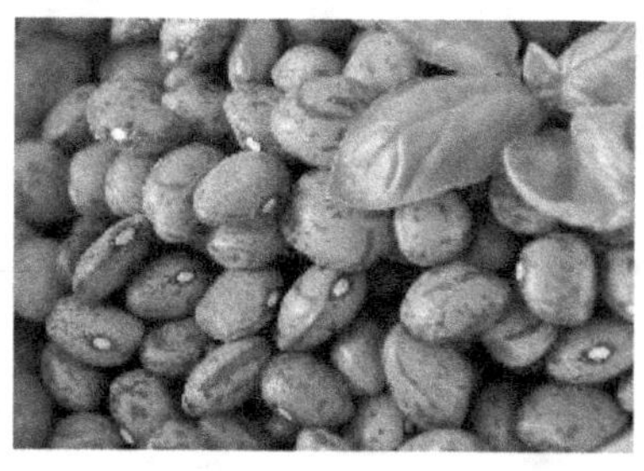

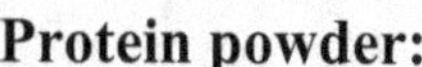

Nuts and nut butters:
Almonds, walnuts, cashews, and peanut butter provide healthy fats and protein for satisfying snacks and meals.

Protein powder:
A convenient option for smoothies, protein shakes, and baking.

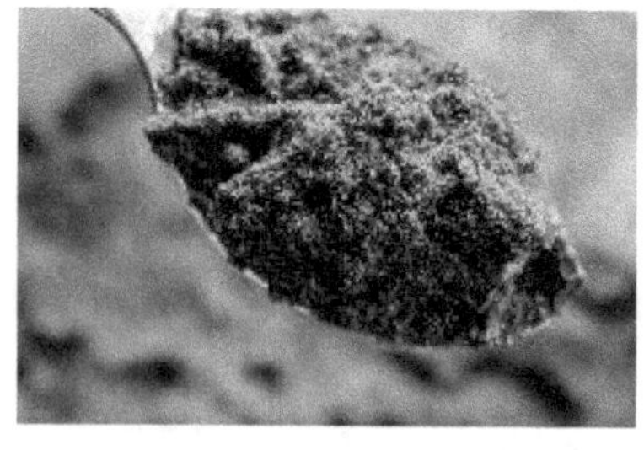

LOW-CARB VEGGIES

Leafy greens:

Spinach, kale, romaine lettuce, arugula, Swiss chard are packed with vitamins and minerals.

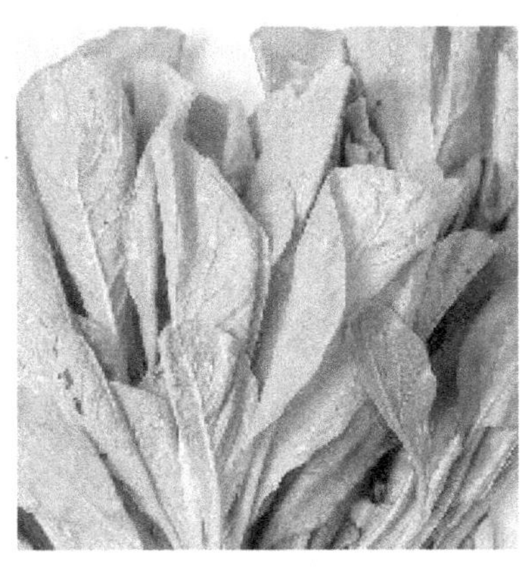

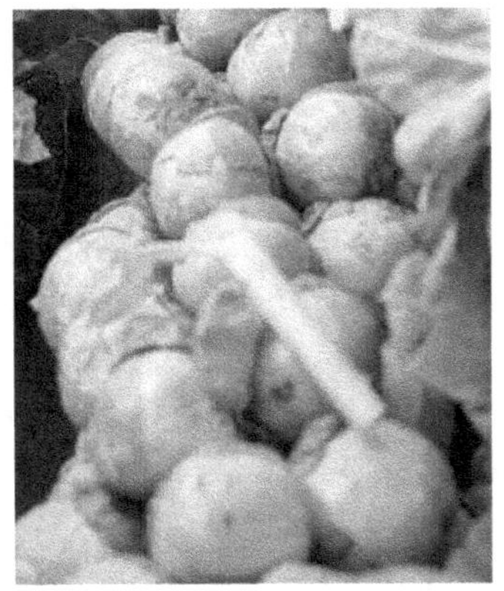

Cruciferous vegetables:
Broccoli, cauliflower, Brussels sprouts, cabbage is high in fiber and offer various health benefits.

Bell peppers:

Available in different colors, offer vitamins, antioxidants, and a sweet flavor.

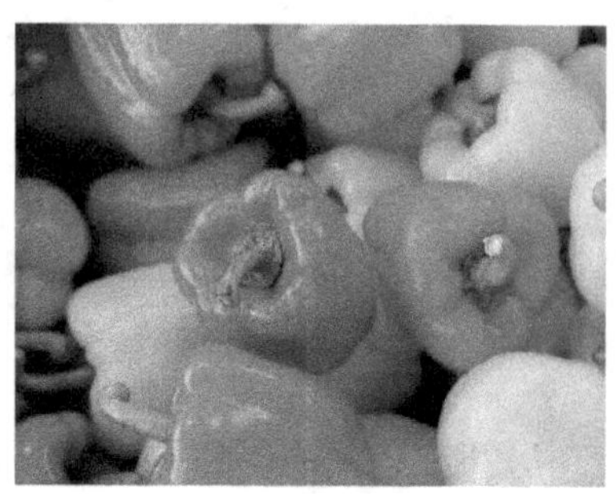

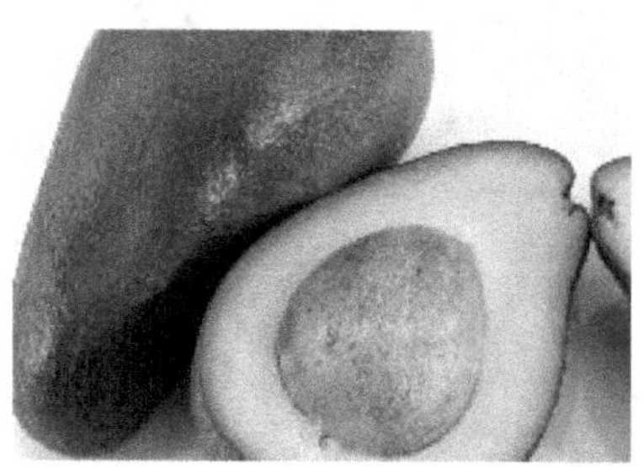

Mushrooms:

Versatile and low in calories, perfect for stir-fries, soups, and omelets.

Avocado:

A healthy fat source with potassium and fiber, perfect for salads, dips, and guacamole.

HEALTHY FATS

Olive oil:

A versatile cooking oil ideal for sautéing, baking, and dressings.

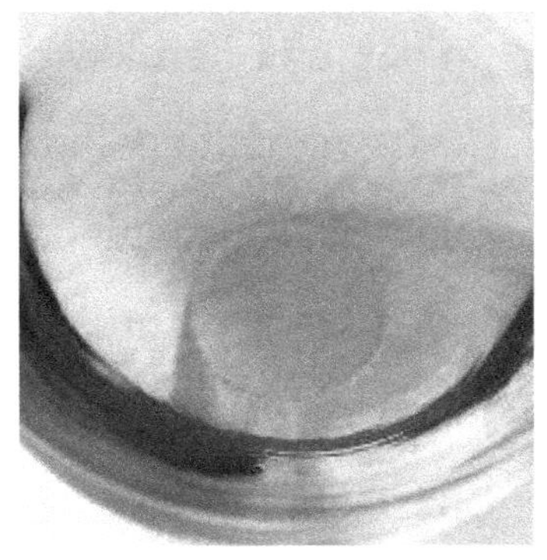

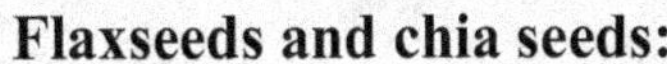

Coconut oil:

A healthy saturated fat with various uses, including cooking, baking, and hair care.

Flaxseeds and chia seeds:
High in fiber and omega-3 fatty acids, great for adding to smoothies, yogurt, or oatmeal.

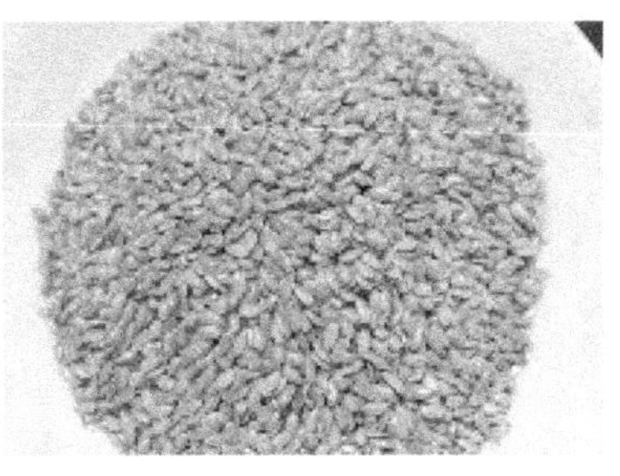

Other Essentials

- **Spices and herbs:** Add flavor and variety to your meals without adding carbs.

- **Sugar-free sweeteners:** Stevia, erythritol, and monk fruit extract are great alternatives for those looking to limit their sugar intake.

- **Unsweetened almond milk and other nut milks:** Low-carb alternatives to dairy milk for coffee, smoothies, and baking.

- **Coconut flour and almond flour:** Low-carb alternatives to wheat flour for baking.

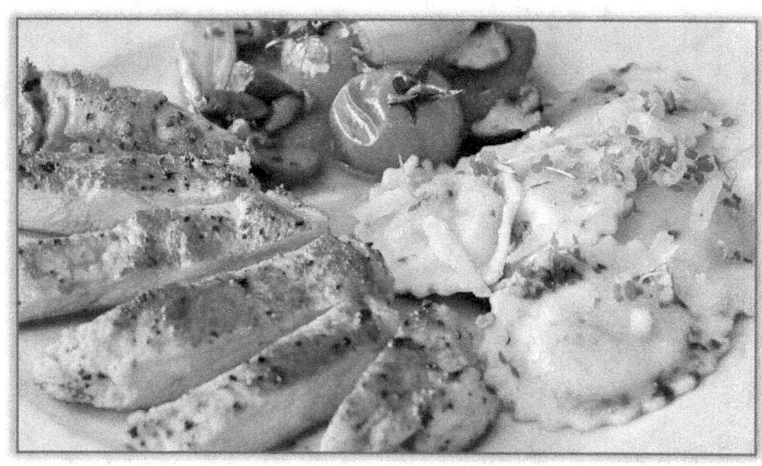

Master Low-Carb, High-Protein Cooking Techniques

Embarking on a low-carb high-protein lifestyle doesn't mean sacrificing deliciousness. With a few simple techniques, you can transform fresh ingredients into flavorful and satisfying meals. Here are some essential cooking techniques to master for your low-carb culinary journey:

1. Sautéing

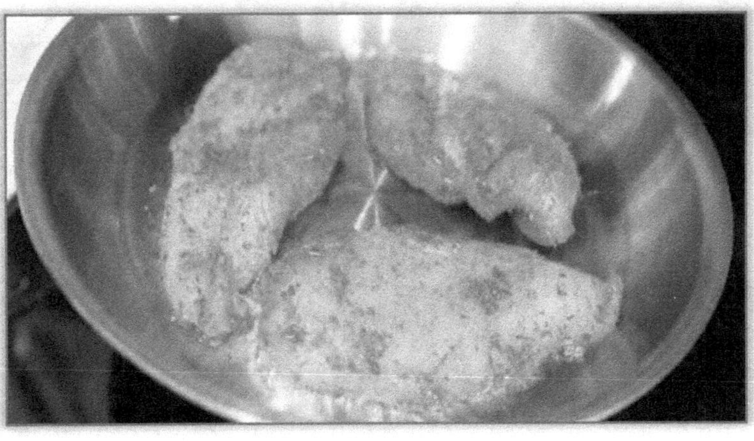

Sautéing involves cooking food quickly in a hot pan with a small amount of oil.

- **Benefits:** Sautéing retains the nutrients and color of vegetables while creating a flavorful sear on meat or fish.

- **Try it with:** Lean meats, chicken breast, fish, shrimp, vegetables like broccoli, asparagus, and bell peppers.

2. Baking

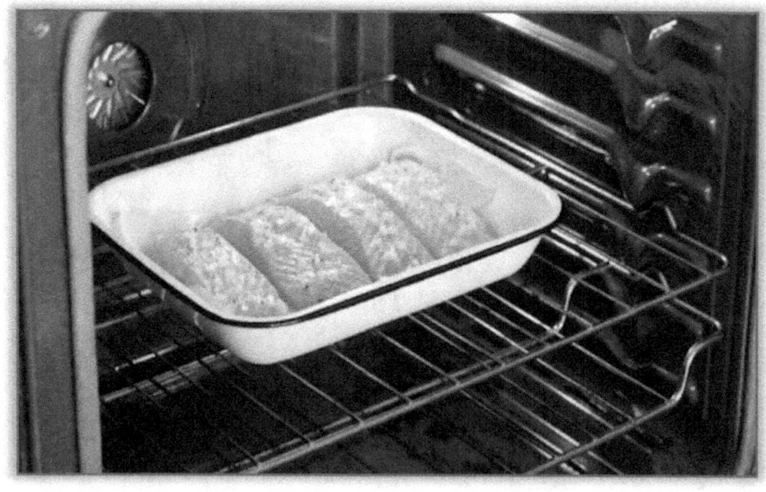

Baking is a versatile cooking method using dry heat to cook food in an oven.

- **Benefits:** Baking retains moisture and nutrients while creating a crispy texture on the outside, ideal for protein and vegetables.

- **Try it with:** Chicken wings, salmon fillets, vegetables like cauliflower, zucchini, and mushrooms.

3. Grilling

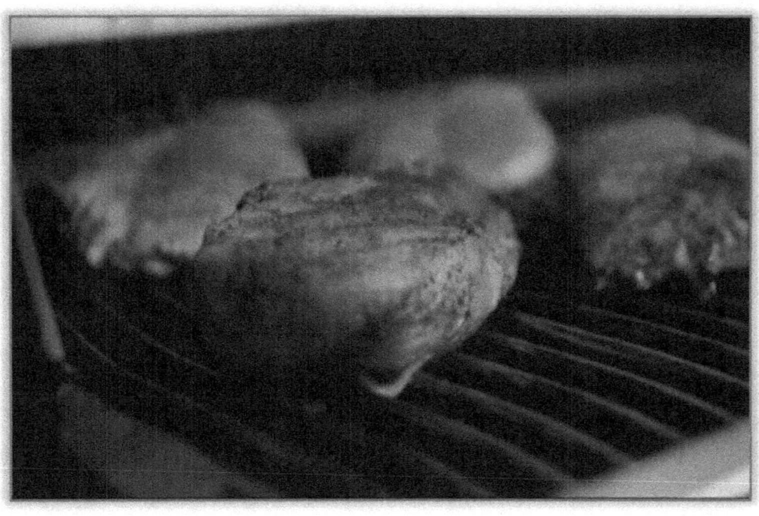

Grilling cooks' food directly over high heat, adding a smoky flavor and crispy texture.

- **Benefits**: Grilling is a healthy cooking method that reduces fat and seals in flavor.
- **Try it with:** Steak, chicken breasts, burgers, vegetables like portobello mushrooms, zucchini slices, and onions.

4. Roasting

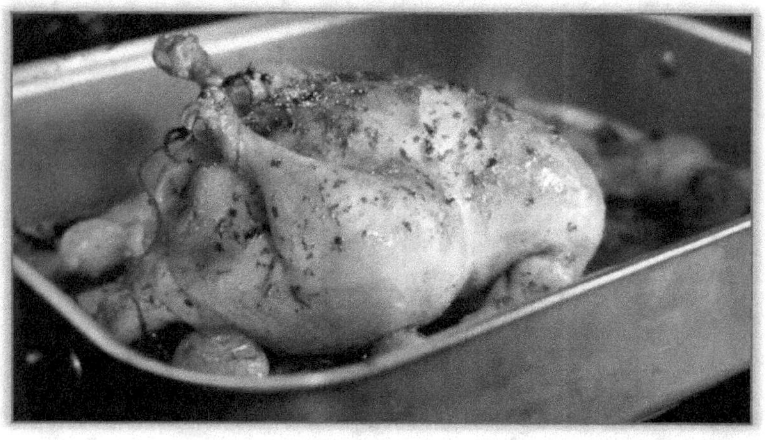

Roasting involves cooking food uncovered in an oven, typically at a high temperature.

- **Benefits:** Roasting caramelizes the exterior of vegetables and meat, creating a rich flavor and tender interior.

- **Try it with:** Whole chickens, pork tenderloin, vegetables like Brussels sprouts, sweet potatoes, and onions.

5. Steaming

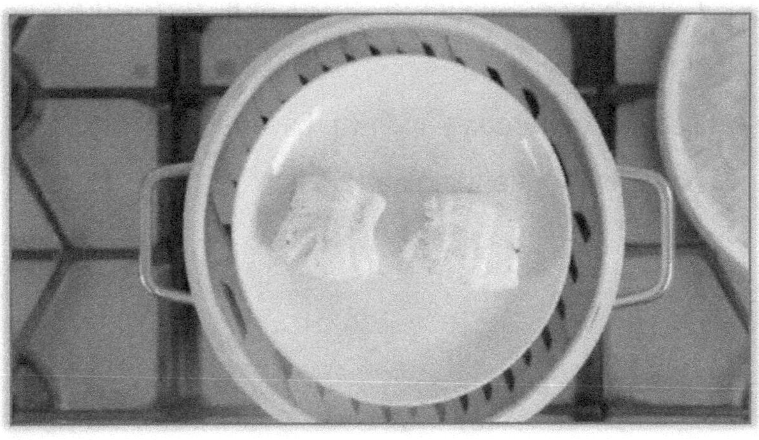

Steaming involves cooking food using the heat from water vapor.

- **Benefits:** Steaming preserves nutrients and moisture, making it a healthy way to cook vegetables and fish.
- **Try it with:** Fish fillets, vegetables like asparagus, broccoli, and green beans.

Bonus Tips:

- Always preheat your pan or oven before adding food.
- Use the right amount of oil to prevent sticking and burning.
- Don't overcook your food to maintain its texture and flavor.
- Season generously with herbs and spices to add flavor without adding carbs.

5 Practical Meal Planning Strategies

A low-carb high-protein diet doesn't have to involve daily culinary acrobatics. With a little planning and preparation, you can create delicious and satisfying meals throughout the week, even amidst busy schedules. some practical tips and strategies include:

1. Start with the Big Picture

- **Set realistic goals**: Don't overwhelm yourself with overly ambitious plans. Start by planning meals for 3-4 days and gradually increase as you get comfortable.

- **Consider dietary needs and preferences:** Are there any allergies or specific dietary restrictions to consider? Plan meals that cater to everyone's needs and preferences.

- **Choose recipes you'll enjoy:** Variety is key to maintaining motivation. Explore different recipes and find dishes you and your family will truly love.

2. **Embrace the Good Prep habits**

- **Batch cook:** Dedicate one day a week to cooking larger batches of protein and vegetables. This saves time throughout the week and provides readily available ingredients for quick and easy meals.

- **Pre-chop vegetables:** Save time and effort by chopping vegetables like onions, peppers, and broccoli in advance and storing them in airtight containers.

3. **Organize Your Kitchen**

- **Invest in storage containers:** Having various sizes of airtight containers allows you to store prepped ingredients and leftovers efficiently.

- **Label everything:** Labeling containers helps you identify ingredients quickly and easily, preventing confusion and waste.

- **Maintain a well-stocked pantry:** Keep essential low-carb high-protein staples like canned tuna, beans, nuts, and protein powder readily available.

4. **Make Meal Planning a Family Activity**

- **Involve everyone:** Encourage family members to participate in meal planning. This creates a sense of ownership and promotes healthy eating habits.

- **Delegate tasks:** Assign simple tasks like washing vegetables or setting the table to younger children, fostering responsibility and teamwork.

5. **Embrace Leftovers**

- **Plan meals with leftovers in mind:** Cook double batches of certain dishes and enjoy them for lunch or dinner the next day.
- **Get creative with leftovers:** Reinvent leftovers into new and exciting dishes. Leftover chicken can be transformed into a salad or sandwich filling, while cooked vegetables can be added to omelets or stir-fries.
- **Freeze portions for future use:** Freeze individual portions of cooked protein and vegetables for busy days or unexpected guests.

Understanding Food Labels

Nutrition Facts

6 servings per container

Serving size   1 cup (65g)

Amount per serving

Calories   230

% Daily Value*

Total Fat 8g	**10%**
Saturated Fat 1g	5%
Trans Fat 0g	
Cholesterol 0mg	**0%**
Sodium 160mg	**7%**
Total Carbohydrate 37g	**13%**
Dietary Fiber 4g	14%
Total Sugars 12g	
Includes 10g Added Sugars	20%
Protein 3g	
Vitamin D 2mcg	10%
Calcium 260mg	20%
Iron 8mg	45%
Potassium 235mg	6%

*The % Daily Value (DV) tells you how much a nutrient in a serving of food contributes to a daily diet. 2,000 calories a day is used for general nutrition advice.

- **Serving Size**

This is the baseline amount of food the manufacturer considers a single serving. Pay attention to the number of servings per container to calculate the total nutrient intake.

- **Calories**

This indicates the total energy provided by a single serving of the food.

- **Total Fat**

This includes all types of fat, including saturated, unsaturated, and trans fats.

- **Saturated and Trans Fats:** Aim to limit these fats, as they can negatively impact your health.
- **Unsaturated Fats:** These are beneficial for your health, so focus on including sources like olive oil, nuts, and avocado.

- **Total Carbohydrates**

This includes all types of carbs, including fiber and sugar.

- **Dietary Fiber:** Fiber such as vegetables, fruits, legumes, and nuts are an important nutrient that contributes to gut health and promotes satiety.
- **Sugars:** This includes naturally occurring sugars and added sugars. Limit your intake of added sugars, as they can contribute to weight gain and other health issues.
- **Protein:** This is a crucial nutrient for building and repairing tissues, maintaining muscle mass, and boosting satiety. Prioritize protein-rich foods like meat, fish, eggs, legumes, and dairy products.

- **Daily Value (%DV)**

This indicates the percentage of the recommended daily intake of a specific nutrient provided by a single serving. This information can help you compare the nutritional value of different products and make informed choices.

Tips for Reading Labels

- **Focus on the carbohydrate content:** Pay attention to the total carbs and sugar content, aiming for options with lower amounts.

- **Choose high-protein foods:** Look for products with at least 20-30% of their calories coming from protein.

- **Be mindful of added sugars:** Limit products with high added sugar content, which contribute to empty calories.

- **Don't be afraid to compare labels:** Compare similar products to choose the option with the most favorable nutritional profile.

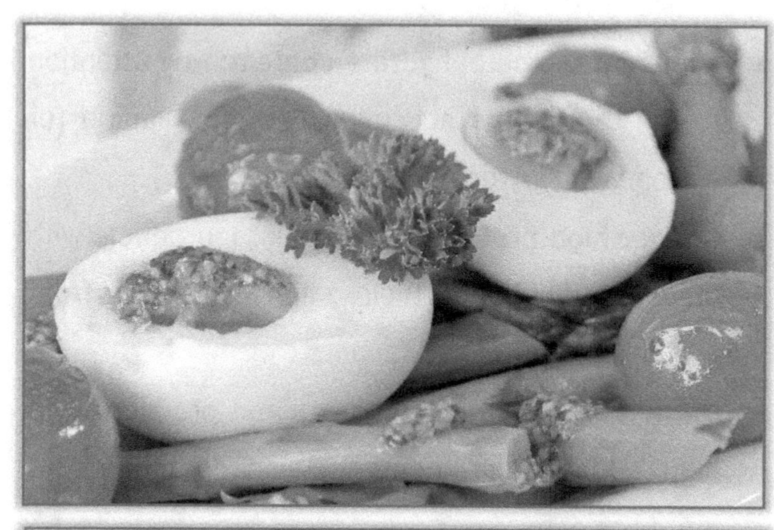

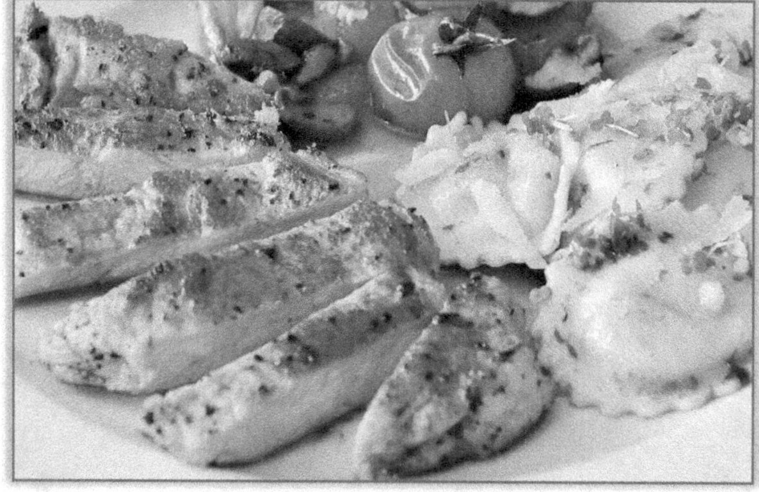

CHAPTER THREE

LOW CARB HIGH PROTEIN RECIPES

Breakfast Meal Plan

Quick & Easy Protein Smoothies

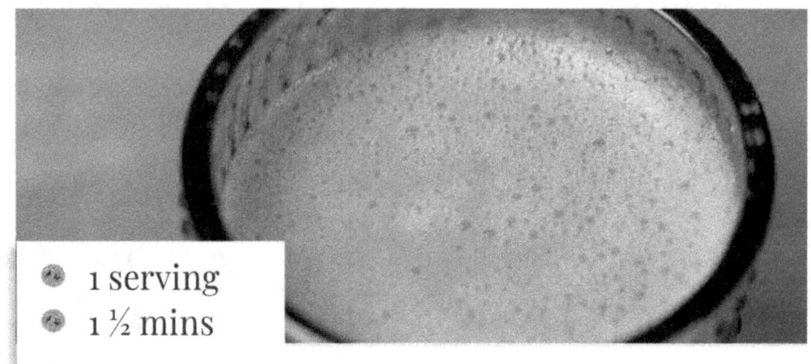

Tropical Green Smoothie

INGREDIENTS

1 cup spinach

1/2 cup frozen pineapple
chunks

1/4 cup frozen mango chunks

1/4 cup plain Greek yogurt

1 scoop protein powder
(vanilla or unflavored)

1/2 cup unsweetened almond
milk

1/4 cup water

Optional: 1 tablespoon chia
seeds or flaxseeds

INSTRUCTIONS

1. Add all ingredients to a
   blender.

2. Blend until smooth and
   creamy.

3. Enjoy immediately!

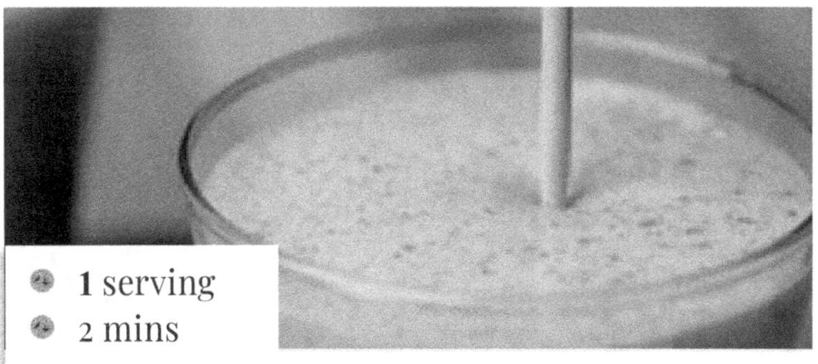

Chocolate Peanut Butter Smoothie

INGREDIENTS

1 cup unsweetened almond milk

1 scoop chocolate protein powder

1/4 cup frozen banana

2 tablespoons natural peanut butter

1/4 cup spinach

1/4 teaspoon ground cinnamon

1/4 teaspoon vanilla extract

Optional: 1/4 cup ice cubes

INSTRUCTIONS

1. Add all ingredients to a blender.
2. Blend until smooth and creamy.
3. Enjoy immediately!

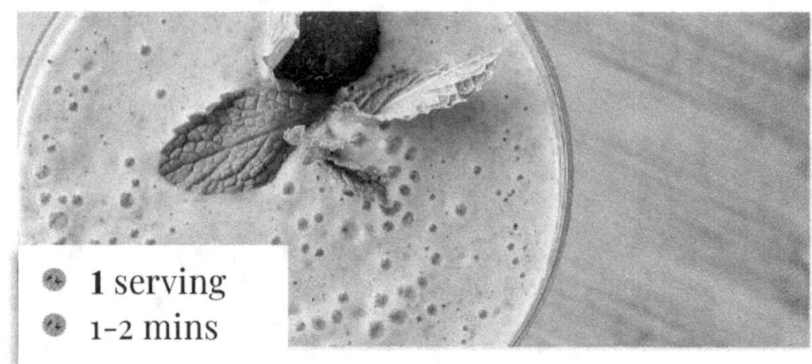

Berry Power Smoothie

INGREDIENTS

1 cup mixed berries
(strawberries, blueberries,
raspberries)
1/2 cup plain Greek yogurt
1/4 cup rolled oats
1 scoop protein powder
(vanilla or unflavored)
1/2 cup unsweetened almond
milk
Optional: 1 tablespoon honey
or maple syrup

INSTRUCTIONS

1. Add all ingredients to a
   blender.
2. Blend until smooth and
   creamy.
3. Enjoy immediately!

Savory Scrambled Eggs

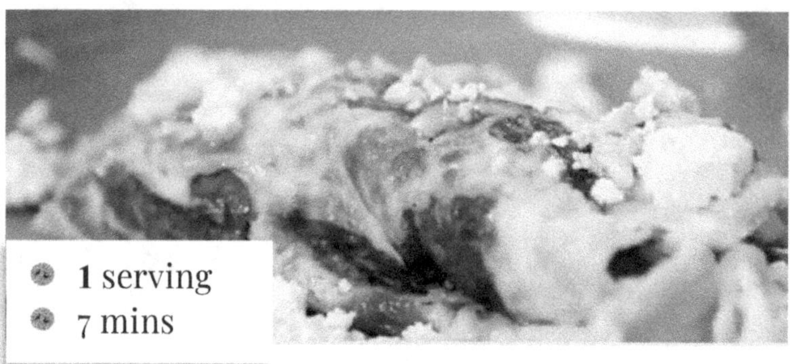

Scrambled Eggs with Spinach and Feta

INGREDIENTS

2 eggs

1 tablespoon olive oil

1/2 cup chopped spinach

1/4 cup crumbled feta cheese

Salt and pepper to taste

INSTRUCTIONS

1. Whisk the eggs in a small bowl.
2. Heat olive oil in a skillet over medium heat.
3. Add the spinach and simmer for about 2 minutes, or until wilted.
4. Add the egg mixture and cook, stirring regularly, until done.
5. Add salt and pepper to taste.
6. Sprinkle with crumbled feta cheese and serve immediately.

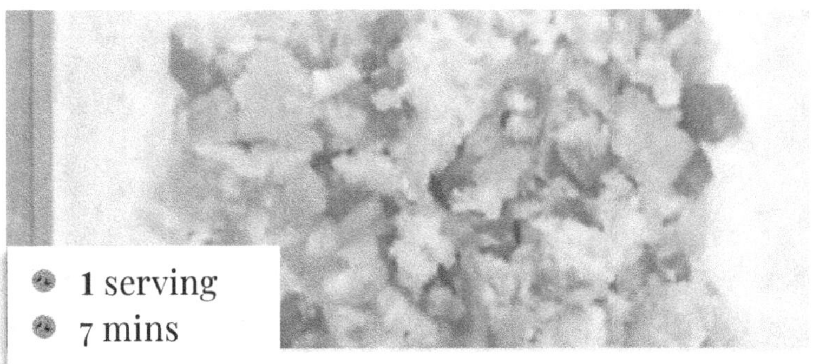

Scrambled Eggs with Ham and Peppers

INGREDIENTS

2 eggs

1 tablespoon olive oil

1/4 cup chopped ham

1/4 cup chopped bell pepper

1/4 cup chopped onion

Salt and pepper to taste

INSTRUCTIONS

1. Whisk the eggs in a small bowl.
2. Heat olive oil in a skillet over medium heat.
3. Add ham, bell pepper, and onion and cook until softened, about 5 minutes.
4. Pour in the egg mixture and cook, stirring frequently, until desired doneness.
5. salt and pepper to taste.
6. Serve immediately.

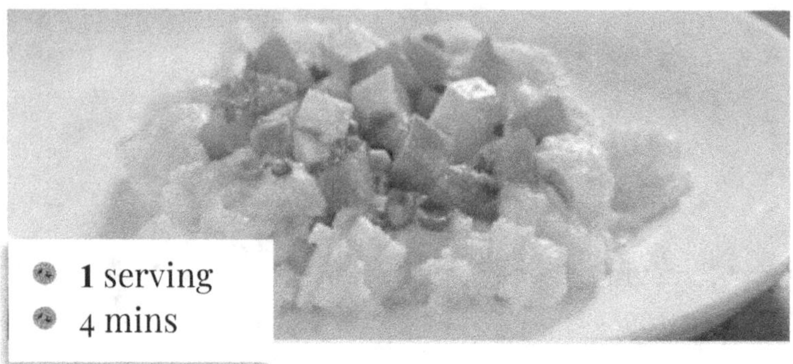

Scrambled Eggs with Avocado Salsa

INGREDIENTS

2 eggs

1 tablespoon olive oil

1/4 cup chopped avocado

Salt and pepper to taste

INSTRUCTIONS

1. Whisk the eggs in a small bowl.
2. Heat olive oil in a skillet over medium heat.
3. Add avocado and cook until softened, about 2 minutes.
4. Pour in the egg mixture and cook, stirring frequently, until desired doneness.
5. Mix chopped avocado with salt and pepper to taste to make salsa.
6. Top with salsa and serve immediately.

Keto Pancakes

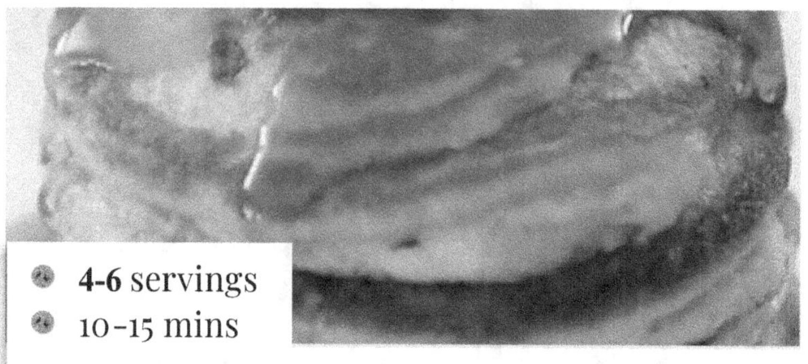

- **4-6** servings
- 10-15 mins

Keto Almond Flour Pancakes

INGREDIENTS

1 cup almond flour

1/4 teaspoon baking powder

1/4 teaspoon salt

1/4 cup unsweetened almond milk

1 egg

1 tablespoon melted coconut oil

1 teaspoon vanilla extract

Optional: Sweetener to taste

INSTRUCTIONS

1. In a large bowl, whisk together almond flour, baking powder, and salt.
2. In a separate bowl, whisk together almond milk, egg, coconut oil, and vanilla extract.
3. Whisk together the wet and dry ingredients until just mixed.
4. Heat a lightly greased griddle or skillet over medium heat.
5. Pour batter onto the griddle, forming pancakes about 4 inches in diameter.
6. Cook for 2-3 minutes per side, or until golden brown.
7. Serve immediately with your favorite toppings.

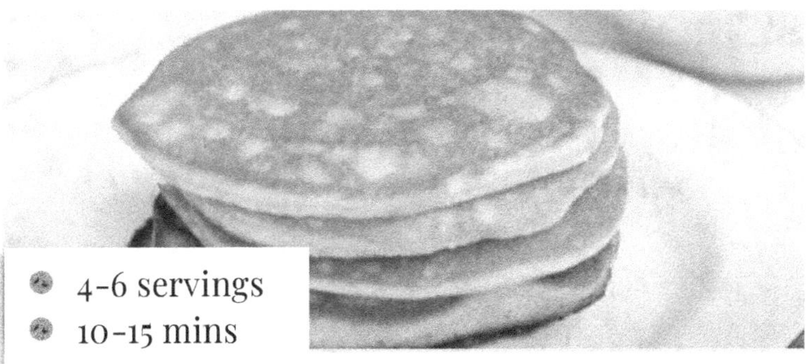

Keto Coconut Flour Pancakes

INGREDIENTS

1/4 cup coconut flour

1/4 cup almond flour

2 teaspoons baking powder

1/4 teaspoon salt

1/4 cup unsweetened almond milk

1 egg

1 tablespoon melted coconut oil

1 teaspoon vanilla extract

Optional: 1/4 cup chopped nuts

Optional: Sweetener to taste

INSTRUCTIONS

1. In a large bowl, whisk together coconut flour, almond flour, baking powder, and salt.
2. In a separate bowl, whisk together almond milk, egg, coconut oil, and vanilla extract.
3. Whisk together the wet and dry ingredients until just mixed.
4. Fold in chopped nuts (if using).
5. Set a lightly greased griddle or skillet over medium heat.
6. Pour batter onto the griddle, forming pancakes about 4 inches in diameter.
7. Cook for 2-3 minutes per side, or until golden brown.
8. Serve immediately with your favorite toppings.

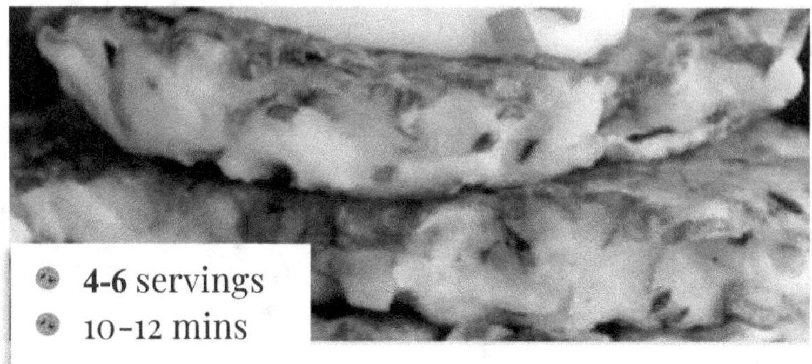

Keto Zucchini Pancakes

INGREDIENTS

1 medium zucchini, grated

1/4 cup almond flour

1/4 cup grated Parmesan cheese

1 egg

1 tablespoon olive oil

1/4 teaspoon salt

1/4 teaspoon black pepper

INSTRUCTIONS

1. Place grated zucchini in a clean dish towel and squeeze out excess moisture.
2. In a large bowl, combine zucchini, almond flour, Parmesan cheese, egg, olive oil, salt, and pepper.
3. Mix well to combine.
4. Heat a lightly greased griddle or skillet over medium heat.
5. Drop zucchini mixture by spoonful onto the griddle, forming small pancakes.
6. Cook for 2-3 minutes per side, or until golden brown.
7. Serve immediately with your favorite toppings.

Overnight Oats

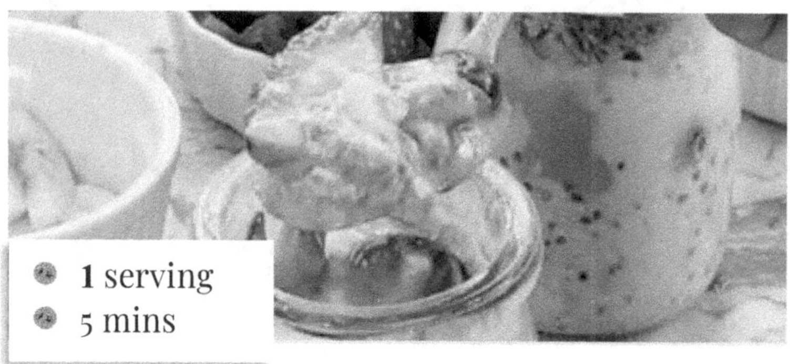

Chia Seed Overnight Oats

INGREDIENTS

1/4 cup rolled oats

2 tablespoons chia seeds

1/2 cup unsweetened almond milk

1/4 cup plain Greek yogurt

1/4 cup berries

1/4 teaspoon vanilla extract

Sweetener to taste (optional)

INSTRUCTIONS

1. In a jar or container with a lid, combine rolled oats, chia seeds, almond milk, Greek yogurt, berries, vanilla extract, and sweetener (if using).
2. Stir well to combine.
3. Cover the jar and refrigerate overnight.
4. In the morning, stir the oats again and add additional toppings such as nuts, seeds, or shredded coconut.
5. Enjoy!

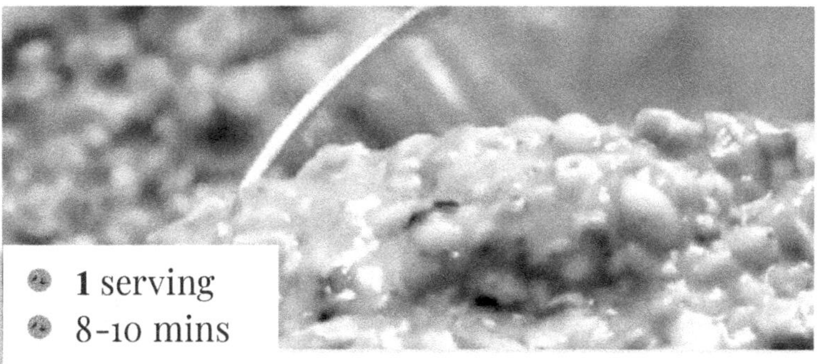

- **1** serving
- 8-10 mins

Keto Overnight Oats

INGREDIENTS

1/4 cup almond flour

1/4 cup coconut flour

1/4 cup chia seeds

1/4 cup unsweetened almond milk

1/4 cup heavy cream

1/4 cup berries

1/4 teaspoon vanilla extract

Sweetener to taste (optional)

INSTRUCTIONS

1. In a jar or container with a lid, combine almond flour, coconut flour, chia seeds, almond milk, heavy cream, berries, vanilla extract, and sweetener (if using).
2. Stir well to combine.
3. Cover the jar and refrigerate overnight.
4. In the morning, stir the oats again and top with additional toppings such as nuts, seeds, or shredded coconut.
5. Enjoy!

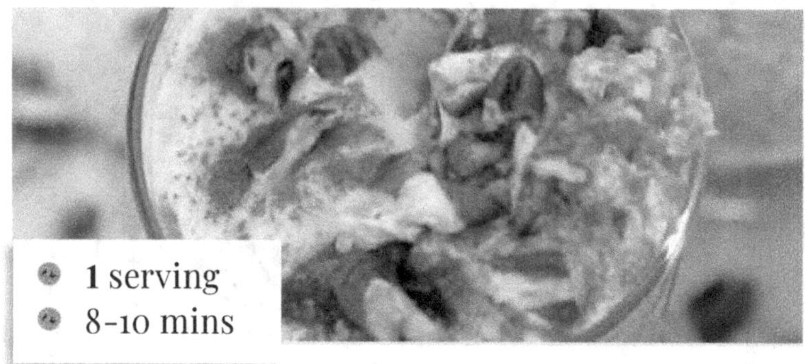

Overnight Oats with Pumpkin

INGREDIENTS

1/4 cup rolled oats

1/4 cup pumpkin puree

1/2 cup unsweetened almond milk

1/4 cup plain Greek yogurt

1/4 cup chopped pecans

1/4 teaspoon cinnamon

Sweetener to taste (optional)

INSTRUCTIONS

1. In a jar or container with a lid, combine rolled oats, pumpkin puree, almond milk, Greek yogurt, pecans, cinnamon, and sweetener (if using).
2. Stir well to combine.
3. Cover the jar and refrigerate overnight.
4. In the morning, stir the oats again and enjoy!

Lunch Meal Plan

Salads & Wraps

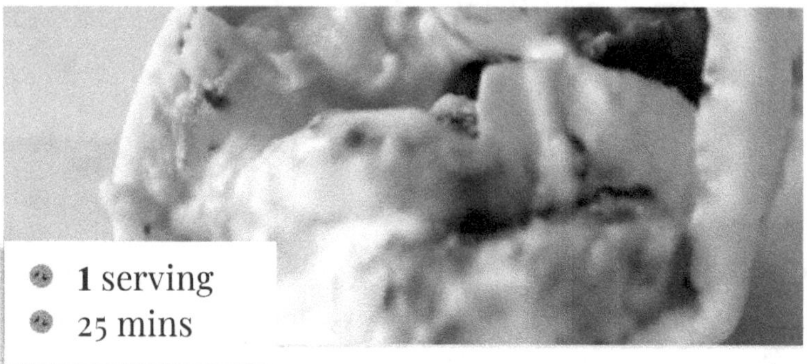

- **1** serving
- 25 mins

Mediterranean Chicken Salad with Hummus Wrap

INGREDIENTS

2 grilled chicken breasts, sliced

1 cup mixed greens

1/2 cup chopped cucumber

1/2 cup chopped tomato

1/4 cup red onion, thinly sliced

1/4 cup crumbled feta cheese

2 tablespoons hummus

1 tablespoon olive oil

1 tablespoon lemon juice

Salt and pepper to taste

INSTRUCTIONS

1. In a bowl, combine chicken, greens, cucumber, tomato, red onion, and feta cheese.
2. In a separate bowl, whisk together hummus, olive oil, lemon juice, salt, and pepper.
3. Spread the hummus mixture on a whole-wheat tortilla.
4. Add the chicken salad mixture to the tortilla.
5. Wrap tightly and enjoy!

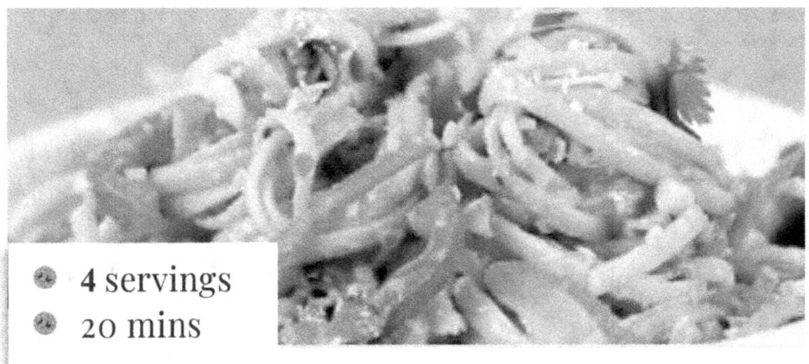

Asian Noodle Salad with Shrimp and Peanut Sauce

INGREDIENTS

1-pound cooked shrimp, peeled and deveined

1 cup cooked rice noodles

1 cup chopped vegetables (e.g., carrots, bell peppers, broccoli)

1/4 cup chopped green onions

1/4 cup chopped peanuts

1/4 cup cilantro, chopped

1/4 cup peanut sauce

INSTRUCTIONS

1. In a large bowl, combine cooked shrimp, rice noodles, vegetables, green onions, peanuts, and cilantro.

2. Toss with peanut sauce and enjoy!

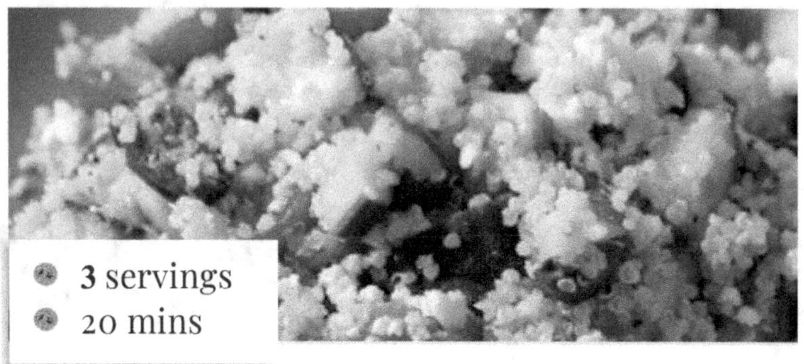

Greek Salad with Quinoa and Lemon Vinaigrette

INGREDIENTS

1 cup cooked quinoa

1 cup chopped romaine lettuce

1/2 cup chopped cucumber

1/2 cup cherry tomatoes, halved

1/4 cup crumbled feta cheese

1/4 cup kalamata olives, pitted and halved

1/4 cup red onion, thinly sliced

1/4 cup olive oil

2 tablespoons lemon juice

1 tablespoon oregano

Salt and pepper to taste

INSTRUCTIONS

1. In a large bowl, combine quinoa, lettuce, cucumber, tomato, feta cheese, olives, and red onion.
2. In a separate bowl, whisk together olive oil, lemon juice, oregano, salt, and pepper.
3. Toss the salad with the dressing until well combined.
4. Serve immediately.

Soups & Stews

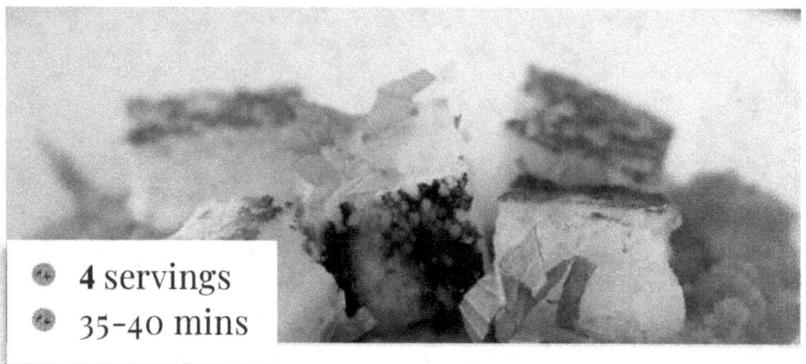

Creamy Tomato Soup with Grilled Cheese Croutons

INGREDIENTS

1 tablespoon olive oil

1 onion, chopped

2 cloves garlic, minced

1 can (28 oz) crushed tomatoes

4 cups chicken broth

1 cup heavy cream

1/4 cup grated Parmesan cheese

1/4 teaspoon dried basil

Salt and pepper to taste

2 slices bread

2 slices cheddar cheese

INSTRUCTIONS

1. Heat olive oil in a large pot over medium heat.
2. Add crushed tomatoes, chicken broth, heavy cream, Parmesan cheese, and basil.
3. Bring to a boil, then reduce heat and simmer for 20 minutes.
4. Meanwhile, butter both sides of the bread slices.
5. Top one slice of bread with cheddar cheese.
6. Place the cheese-topped bread on top of the other slice of bread, forming a sandwich.
7. Heat a skillet over medium heat and cook the sandwich until golden brown on both sides.
8. Cut the sandwich into cubes and set aside.
9. Puree the soup with an immersion blender or in batches in a blender.
10. Season with salt and pepper to taste. Serve soup.

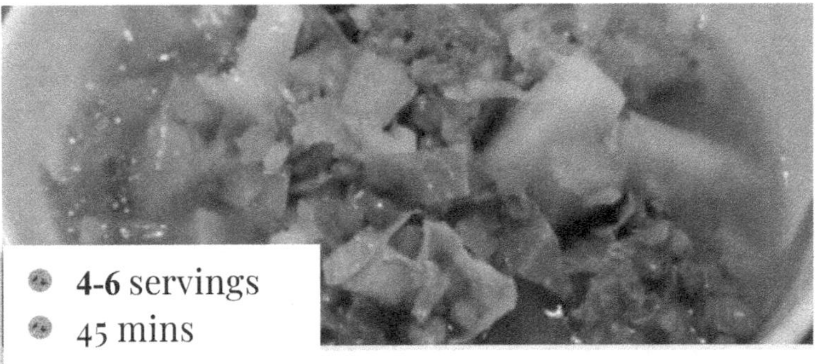

Lentil Soup with Smoked Sausage

INGREDIENTS

1 tablespoon olive oil

1 onion, chopped

2 carrots, chopped

2 celery stalks, chopped

2 cloves garlic, minced

1 cup lentils, rinsed

4 cups chicken broth

1 cup chopped smoked sausage

1/4 cup chopped fresh parsley

Salt and pepper to taste

INSTRUCTIONS

1. add the olive oil in a big pot or Dutch oven over medium heat.
2. Cook the onion, carrots, celery, and garlic for 5 minutes, or until softened.
3. Add lentils, chicken broth, smoked sausage, and 1/2 cup of parsley.
4. Bring to a boil, then reduce heat and simmer for 20-25 minutes, or until lentils are tender.
5. salt and pepper to taste.
6. Serve hot, garnished with remaining parsley.

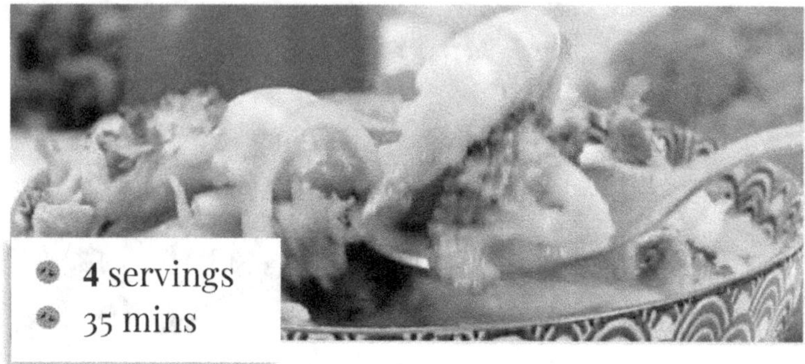

Thai Coconut Curry Soup with Shrimp

INGREDIENTS

1 tablespoon olive oil

1 onion, chopped

2 cloves garlic, minced

1 tablespoon red curry paste

1 can (14 oz) coconut milk

4 cups chicken broth

1-pound shrimp, peeled and deveined

1/2 cup chopped bell peppers

1/4 cup chopped cilantro

1 tablespoon lime juice

1 tablespoon fish sauce

Salt and pepper to taste

INSTRUCTIONS

1. add olive oil in a large pot or Dutch oven over medium heat.
2. Cook the onion for 5 minutes, or until softened.
3. Add garlic and red curry paste and cook for another minute.
4. Add coconut milk, chicken broth, shrimp, bell peppers, and 1/2 cup of cilantro.
5. Bring to a boil, then reduce heat and simmer for 10-15 minutes, or until shrimp are cooked through.
6. Stir in lime juice and fish sauce.
7. Season with salt and pepper to taste.
8. Serve hot, garnished with remaining cilantro.

Sandwich Alternatives

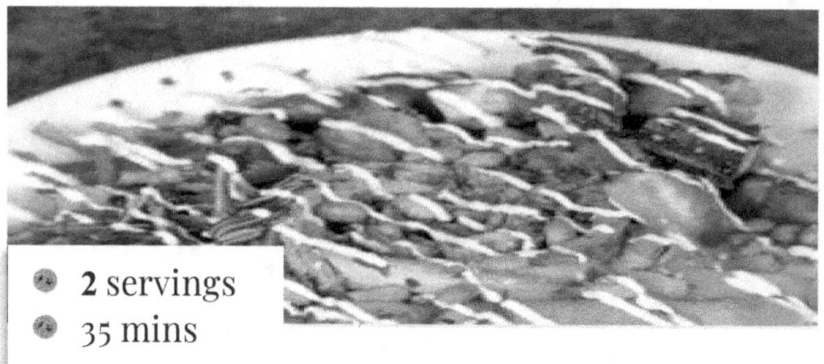

Salmon Sushi Bowls with Brown Rice and Avocado

INGREDIENTS

1 cup cooked rice

1 cup cooked salmon, flaked

1/2 cup chopped cucumber

1/2 cup chopped avocado

1/4 cup pickled ginger

1/4 cup seaweed salad

1 tablespoon soy sauce

1 tablespoon sesame oil

1 tablespoon rice vinegar

1 teaspoon sriracha (optional)

Sesame seeds, for garnish

INSTRUCTIONS

1. Divide the rice among bowls.
2. Top with salmon, cucumber, avocado, pickled ginger, and seaweed salad.
3. In a small bowl, whisk together soy sauce, sesame oil, rice vinegar, and sriracha (if using).
4. Drizzle the dressing over the bowls.
5. Garnish with sesame seeds and enjoy!

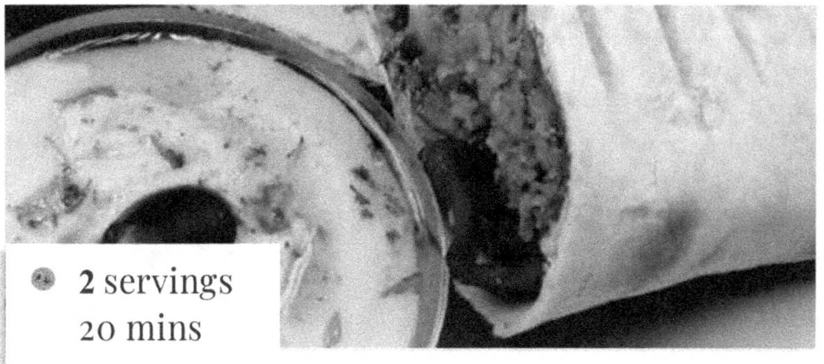

Veggie Wraps with Hummus and Tahini Dressing

INGREDIENTS

2 whole wheat tortillas

1/2 cup hummus

1/4 cup tahini dressing

1 cup mixed greens

1/2 cup chopped cucumber

1/2 cup chopped bell

peppers

1/4 cup crumbled feta

cheese

Fresh herbs, such as

parsley or cilantro

(optional)

INSTRUCTIONS

1. Spread hummus on each tortilla.
2. Drizzle with tahini dressing.
3. Top with mixed greens, cucumber, bell peppers, and feta cheese.
4. Add fresh herbs (if using).
5. Roll tightly and enjoy!

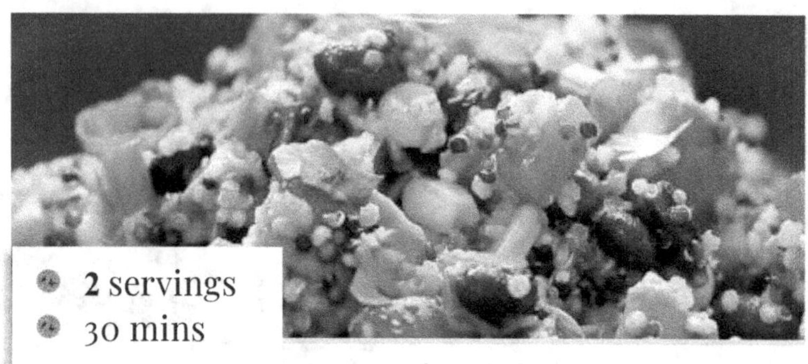

Quinoa Power Bowls with Black Beans and Roasted Vegetables

INGREDIENTS

1 cup cooked quinoa

1 cup cooked black beans

1 cup roasted vegetables

(e.g., broccoli, carrots,

onions)

1/4 cup chopped avocado

1/4 cup chopped fresh

cilantro

1/4 cup lime crema

(optional)

1 tablespoon olive oil

1 tablespoon lime juice

Salt and pepper to taste

INSTRUCTIONS

1. Divide the quinoa and black beans among bowls.
2. Top with roasted vegetables, avocado, and cilantro.
3. Drizzle with lime crema (if using).
4. In a small bowl, whisk together olive oil, lime juice, salt, and pepper.
5. Drizzle the dressing over the bowls.
6. Serve immediately.

Buddha Bowls

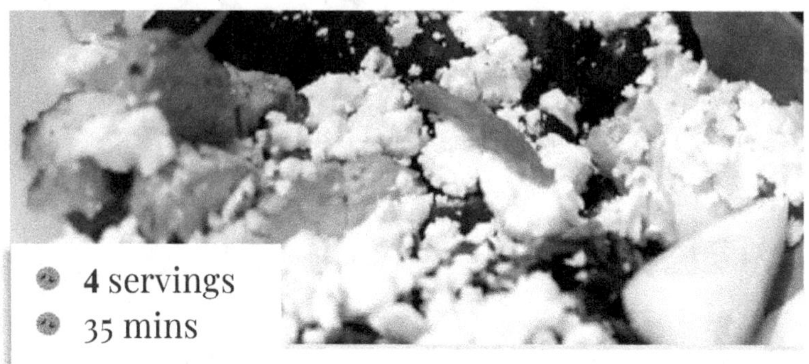

- **4** servings
- 35 mins

Mediterranean Buddha Bowl with Chicken and Feta

INGREDIENTS

1 cup cooked quinoa
1 cup grilled chicken, chopped
1 cup chopped romaine lettuce
1/2 cup chopped cucumber
1/2 cup chopped cherry tomatoes
1/4 cup crumbled feta cheese
1/4 cup pitted kalamata olives
1/4 cup red onion, thinly sliced
1/4 cup hummus
2 tablespoons olive oil
1 tablespoon lemon juice
Salt and pepper to taste

INSTRUCTIONS

1. Divide the quinoa among bowls.
2. Top with chicken, romaine lettuce, cucumber, cherry tomatoes, feta cheese, olives, and red onion.
3. Drizzle with hummus.
4. In a small bowl, whisk together olive oil, lemon juice, salt, and pepper.
5. Drizzle the dressing over the bowls.
6. Serve immediately.

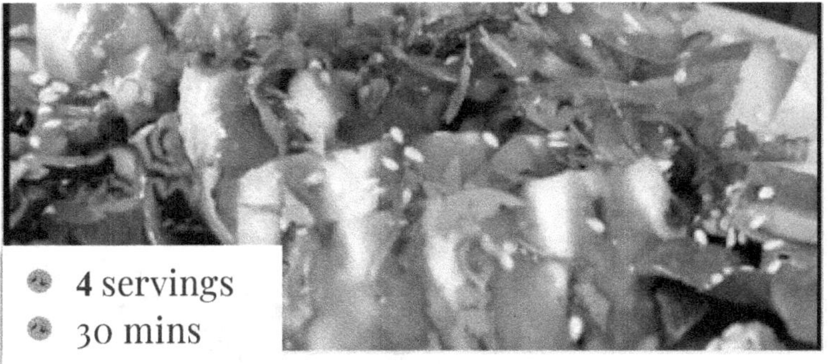

<u>*Thai Buddha Bowl with Tofu and Peanut Sauce*</u>

- **4** servings
- 30 mins

INGREDIENTS

1 cup cooked brown rice

1 cup cooked tofu, cubed and pan-fried

1 cup chopped vegetables (e.g., broccoli, carrots, bell peppers)

1/2 cup chopped mango

1/4 cup chopped red onion

1/4 cup chopped peanuts

1/4 cup cilantro, chopped

1/4 cup peanut sauce

INSTRUCTIONS

1. Divide the brown rice among bowls.
2. Top with tofu, vegetables, mango, red onion, peanuts, and cilantro.
3. Drizzle with peanut sauce.
4. Serve immediately.

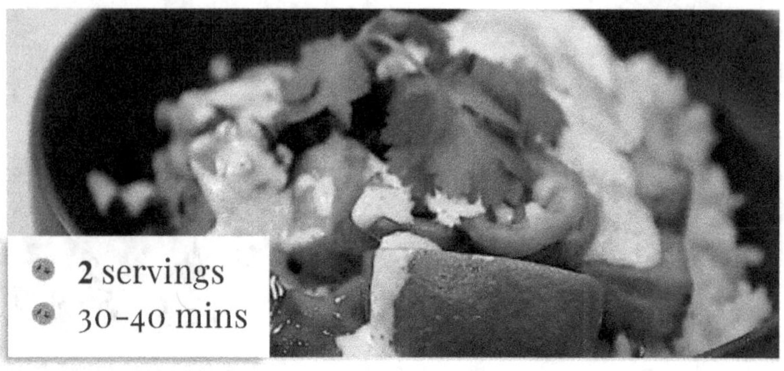

Detox Buddha Bowl with Black Beans and Sweet Potato

INGREDIENTS

1 cup cooked quinoa

1 cup cooked black beans

1 roasted sweet potato, diced

1 cup chopped kale

1/2 cup chopped avocado

1/4 cup chopped red onion

1/4 cup chopped cilantro

1 tablespoon olive oil

1 tablespoon lemon juice

1/2 teaspoon cumin

Salt and pepper to taste

INSTRUCTIONS

1. Divide the quinoa and black beans among bowls.
2. Top with roasted sweet potato, kale, avocado, and red onion.
3. Sprinkle with cilantro.
4. Mix together olive oil, lemon juice, cumin, salt, and pepper.
5. Drizzle the dressing over the bowls.
6. Serve immediately.

Dinner Meal Plan

One-Pan Meals

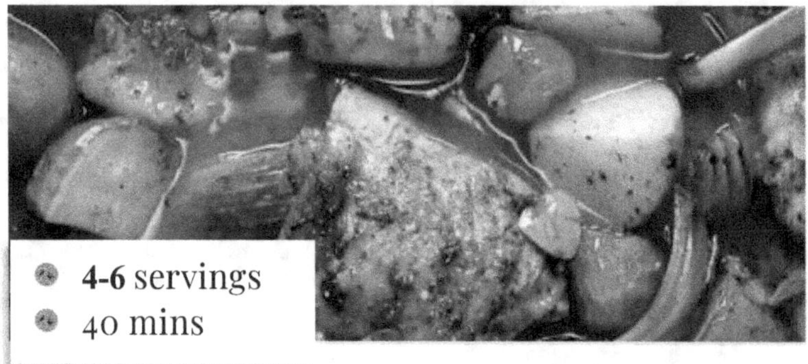

Lemon Garlic Chicken with Roasted Vegetables

<table>
<tr><td valign="top" width="50%">

INGREDIENTS

2 pounds boneless,

skinless chicken breasts

2 tablespoons olive oil

1 tablespoon lemon juice

1 tablespoon garlic

powder

1 teaspoon dried oregano

1/2 teaspoon salt

1/4 teaspoon black pepper

1 cup chopped carrots

1 cup chopped broccoli

florets

1/2 cup chopped red onion

</td><td valign="top" width="50%">

INSTRUCTIONS

7. Preheat oven to 400°F (200°C).
8. In a bowl, whisk together olive oil, lemon juice, garlic powder, oregano, salt, and pepper.
9. Place chicken breasts in a baking dish and coat with the marinade.
10. Add carrots, broccoli, and red onion to the baking dish.
11. Toss to coat the vegetables with the marinade.
12. Bake for 25-30 minutes, or until chicken is cooked through and vegetables are tender.
13. Serve immediately.

</td></tr>
</table>

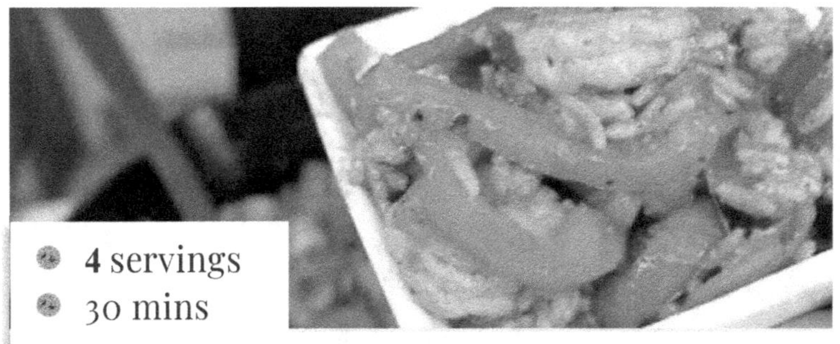

Sausage and Peppers with Rice

INGREDIENTS

1-pound Italian sausage links, sliced

1 tablespoon olive oil

1 onion, chopped

2 bell peppers, chopped

1 cup uncooked long-grain white rice

2 cups chicken broth

1/2 teaspoon dried thyme

1/4 cup chopped fresh parsley

Salt and pepper to taste

INSTRUCTIONS

1. Heat olive oil in a large skillet over medium heat.
2. cook sausage until browned, about 5 minutes.
3. Add and cook onion until softened, about 5 minutes.
4. Add bell peppers and cook until tender-crisp, about 5 minutes.
5. Stir in rice, chicken broth, thyme, salt, and pepper.
6. Bring to a boil, then reduce heat and simmer for 20-25 minutes, or until rice is cooked through and liquid is absorbed.
7. Fluff with a fork and stir in parsley.
8. Serve immediately.

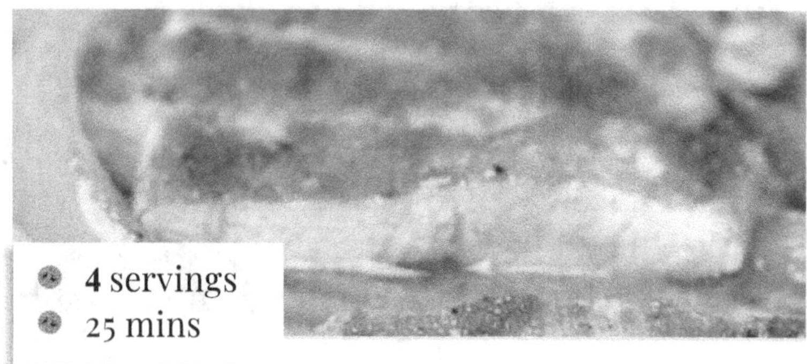

Sheet Pan Fajitas

INGREDIENTS

1-pound boneless, skinless chicken breasts, sliced

1 bell pepper, sliced

1 onion, sliced

1/2 cup fajita seasoning

1/4 cup olive oil

1 tablespoon lime juice

Warm tortillas

Fajita toppings (e.g., salsa, guacamole, sour cream)

INSTRUCTIONS

1. Preheat oven to 400°F (200°C).
2. In a bowl, toss chicken, bell pepper, onion, fajita seasoning, olive oil, and lime juice.
3. Spread the mixture onto a baking sheet.
4. Bake for 20-25 minutes, or until chicken is cooked through and vegetables are tender.
5. Serve immediately with warm tortillas and desired fajita toppings.

Slow Cooker & Instant Pot Recipes

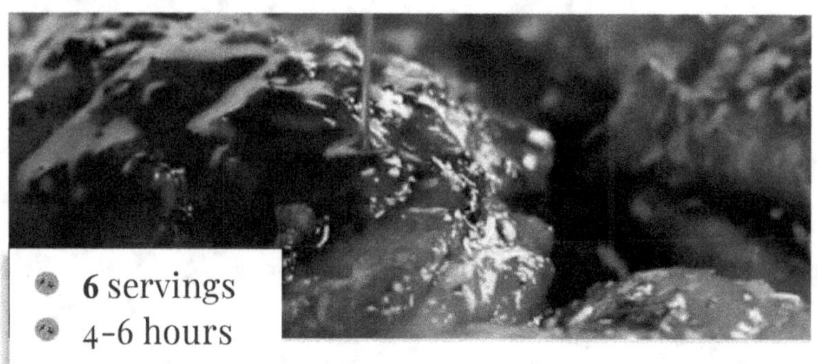

Slow Cooker Honey Garlic Chicken

INGREDIENTS

2 pounds boneless, skinless chicken thighs

1/2 cup honey

1/4 cup soy sauce

1 tablespoon rice vinegar

1 tablespoon cornstarch

1 tablespoon minced ginger

1 clove garlic, minced

1/2 teaspoon red pepper flakes (optional)

INSTRUCTIONS

1. Combine all ingredients in a slow cooker.
2. Cook for 6-8 hours, or 3-4 hours, on low or high.
3. Shred chicken with two forks.
4. Serve over rice or noodles.

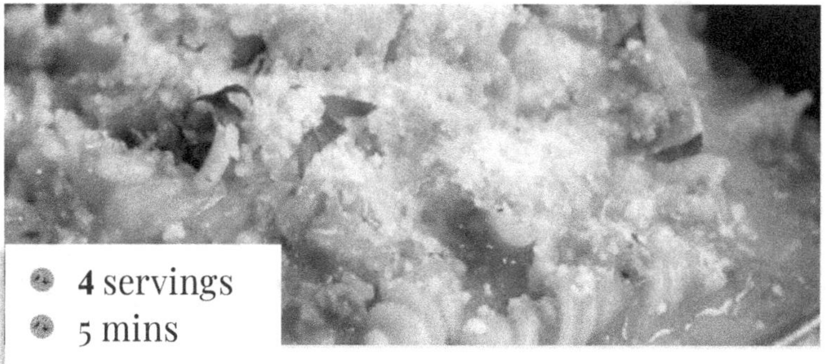

Instant Pot Creamy Tomato Pasta

INGREDIENTS

1-pound ground beef

1 onion, chopped

2 cloves garlic, minced

1 (28-ounce) can crushed tomatoes

1 cup beef broth

1/2 cup heavy cream

1/4 cup grated Parmesan cheese

1 teaspoon dried oregano

1/2 teaspoon salt

1/4 teaspoon black pepper

12 ounces dried pasta

INSTRUCTIONS

1. Turn on sauté mode on the Instant Pot.
2. Add ground beef, onion, and garlic and cook until browned.
3. Add crushed tomatoes, beef broth, heavy cream, Parmesan cheese, oregano, salt, and pepper.
4. Stir in pasta.
5. Pressure cook on for 4 minutes.
6. Allow natural release for 5 minutes, then release remaining pressure manually.
7. Stir in pasta and cook until heated through.
8. Serve immediately.

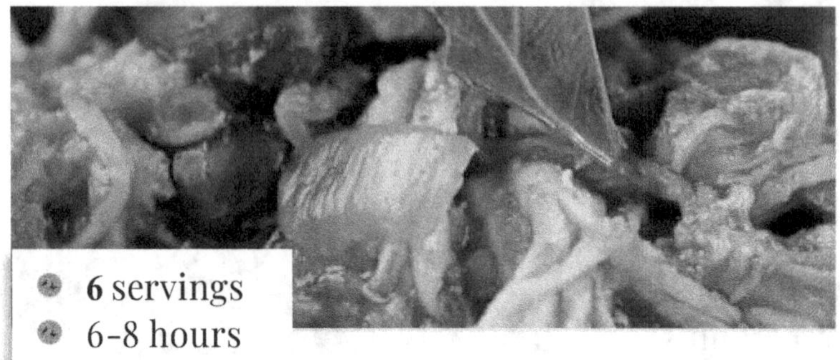

Slow Cooker Chicken Chili

INGREDIENTS

2 pounds boneless, skinless chicken thighs, chopped

1 onion, chopped

2 cloves garlic, minced

1 (15-ounce) can diced tomatoes, undrained

1 (15-ounce) rinsed and drained can kidney beans.

1 (15-ounce) rinsed and drained can black beans

1 cup chicken broth

1 tablespoon chili powder

1 teaspoon cumin

1/2 teaspoon dried oregano

1/2 teaspoon salt

1/4 teaspoon black pepper

INSTRUCTIONS

1. Combine all ingredients in a slow cooker.
2. Cook for 6-8 hours, or 3-4 hours, low or high.
3. Serve with desired toppings, such as sour cream, shredded cheese, and avocado.

Stir-Fries & Sautés

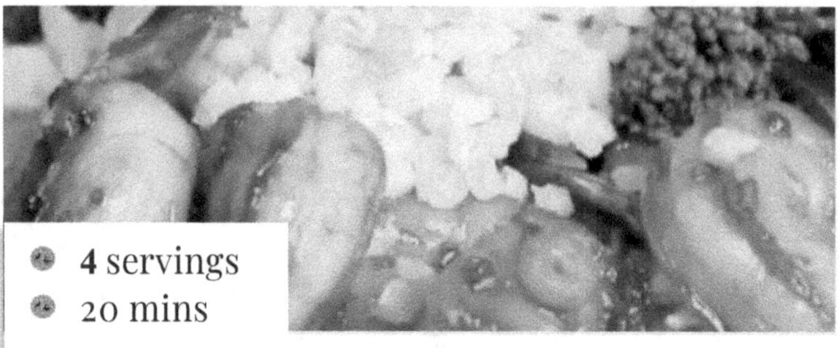

Honey Garlic Shrimp Stir-Fry

INGREDIENTS

1-pound shrimp, peeled and deveined

1 tablespoon cornstarch

1 tablespoon olive oil

1 onion, chopped

2 cloves garlic, minced

1 bell pepper, sliced

1/2 cup honey

1/4 cup soy sauce

1 tablespoon rice vinegar

1 tablespoon sriracha (optional)

Cooked rice or noodles

INSTRUCTIONS

1. Toss shrimp in cornstarch.
2. Add olive oil in a large skillet or wok over medium-high heat.
3. Add shrimp and cook until pink and cooked through, about 3 minutes.
4. Remove shrimp from the pan and set aside.
5. Add onion and garlic to the pan and cook until softened, about 5 minutes.
6. Add bell pepper and cook until tender-crisp, about 5 minutes.
7. Stir in honey, soy sauce, rice vinegar, and sriracha (if using).
8. Add shrimp back to the pan and cook until heated through.
9. Serve over rice or noodles.

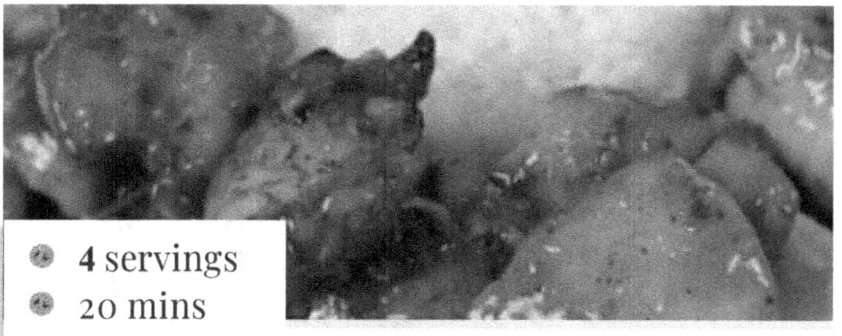

Chicken Teriyaki Stir-Fry

INGREDIENTS

1 pound boneless, skinless chicken breasts, sliced

1 tablespoon cornstarch

1 tablespoon olive oil

1 onion, chopped

2 cloves garlic, minced

1 bell pepper, sliced

1/2 cup teriyaki sauce

1/4 cup pineapple chunks

1 tablespoon sesame oil

Cooked rice or noodles

INSTRUCTIONS

1. Toss chicken in cornstarch.
2. add olive oil in a large skillet or wok over medium-high heat.
3. Add chicken and cook until browned and cooked through, about 5 minutes.
4. Remove chicken from the pan and set aside.
5. Add onion and garlic to the pan and cook until softened, about 5 minutes.
6. Add bell pepper and cook until tender-crisp, about 5 minutes.
7. Stir in teriyaki sauce and pineapple chunks.
8. Add chicken back to the pan and cook until heated through.
9. Stir in sesame oil.
10. 10. Serve over rice or noodles.

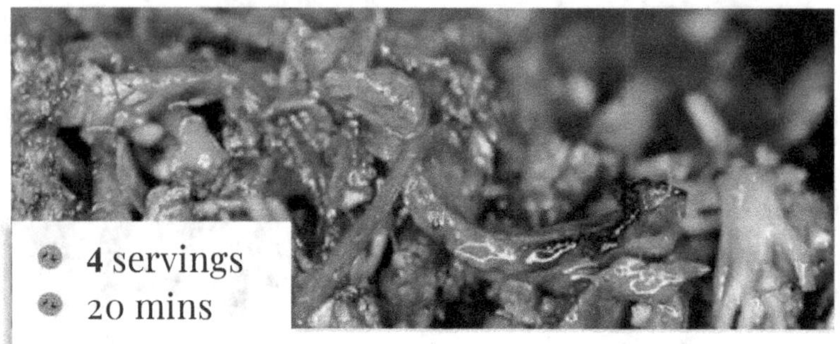

Beef and Broccoli Stir-Fry

INGREDIENTS

1 pound flank steak, thinly sliced

1 tablespoon cornstarch

1 tablespoon olive oil

1 onion, chopped

2 cloves garlic, minced

1 head broccoli, cut into florets

1/2 cup soy sauce

1/4 cup brown sugar

1 tablespoon rice vinegar

1 teaspoon sriracha (optional)

Cooked rice or noodles

INSTRUCTIONS

1. Toss flank steak in cornstarch.
2. add olive oil in a large skillet or wok over medium-high heat.
3. Add flank steak and cook until browned and cooked through, about 5 minutes.
4. Remove flank steak from the pan and set aside.
5. Add onion and garlic to the pan and cook until softened, about 5 minutes.
6. Add broccoli and cook until tender-crisp, about 5 minutes.
7. Stir in soy sauce, brown sugar, rice vinegar, and sriracha (if using).
8. Add flank steak back to the pan and cook until heated through.
9. Serve over rice or noodles.

Stuffed Vegetables & Meatballs

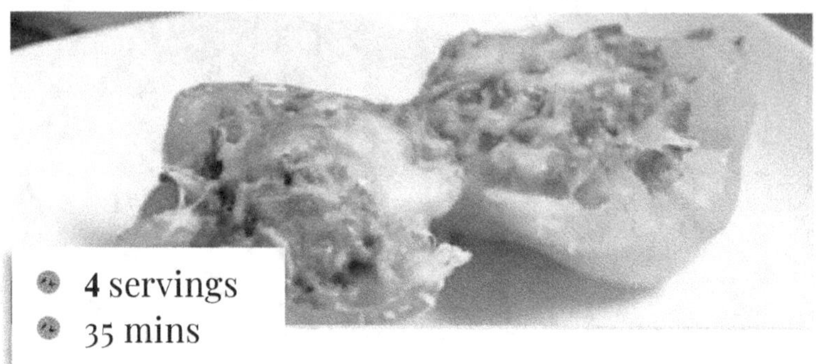

- **4** servings
- 35 mins

Stuffed Peppers with Ground Beef and Rice

INGREDIENTS

4 bell peppers

1 pound ground beef

1/2 cup chopped onion

1/2 cup chopped celery

1/2 cup cooked rice

1/4 cup chopped fresh parsley

1/4 cup tomato sauce

1 tablespoon Worcestershire sauce

1 teaspoon salt

1/2 teaspoon black pepper

INSTRUCTIONS

1. Preheat oven to 375°F (190°C).
2. Cut tops off peppers and remove seeds and membranes.
3. Cook ground beef, onion, and celery in a large skillet over medium heat until browned.
4. Drain any excess fat.
5. Stir in rice, parsley, tomato sauce, Worcestershire sauce, salt, and pepper.
6. Fill peppers with the mixture.
7. Place peppers in a baking dish and add 1/2 inch of water to the bottom of the dish.
8. Bake for 30-35 minutes, or until peppers are tender.
9. Serve immediately.

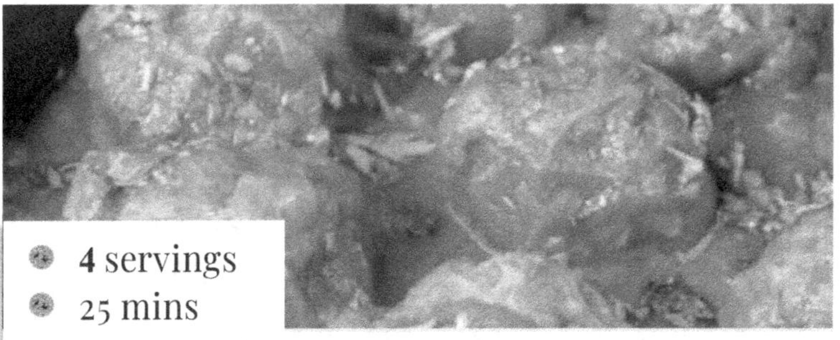

Turkey Meatballs with Marinara Sauce

INGREDIENTS

1 pound ground turkey
1/2 cup bread crumbs
1/4 cup grated Parmesan cheese
1/4 cup chopped fresh parsley
1 egg
1 tablespoon olive oil
1 (28-ounce) can crushed tomatoes
1 tablespoon dried oregano
1 teaspoon garlic powder
1/2 teaspoon salt
1/4 teaspoon black pepper

INSTRUCTIONS

1. Preheat oven to 400°F (200°C).
2. In a large bowl, combine ground turkey, bread crumbs, Parmesan cheese, parsley, egg, olive oil, oregano, garlic powder, salt, and pepper.
3. Mix well and form into balls.
4. Place meatballs on a baking sheet and bake for 20-25 minutes, or until cooked through.
5. While the meatballs are baking, heat crushed tomatoes in a saucepan over medium heat.
6. Serve meatballs with marinara sauce.

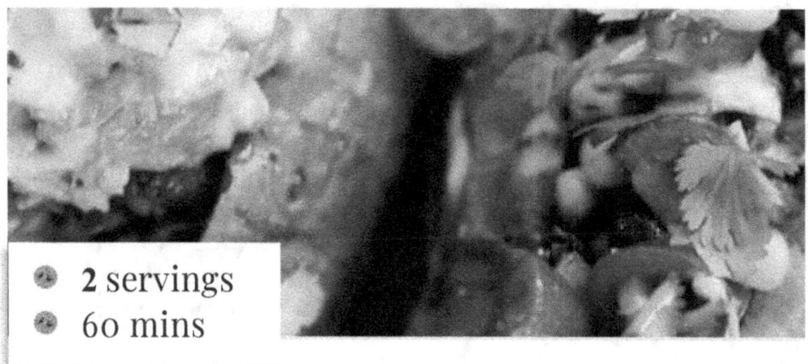

- **2** servings
- 60 mins

Stuffed Sweet Potatoes with Black Beans and Corn

INGREDIENTS

2 large sweet potatoes
1 tablespoon olive oil
1 onion, chopped
1 red bell pepper, chopped
1 clove garlic, minced
1 (15-ounce) drained and rinsed can black beans,
1/2 cup frozen corn
1/4 cup chopped fresh cilantro
1 tablespoon lime juice
1/2 teaspoon cumin
1/4 teaspoon chili powder
Salt and pepper to taste

INSTRUCTIONS

1. Preheat oven to 400°F (200°C).
2. Pierce sweet potatoes with a fork and bake for 45-60 minutes, or until tender.
3. Heat olive oil in a large skillet over medium heat.
4. Add onion and bell pepper and cook until softened, about 5 minutes.
5. Add garlic, black beans, corn, cilantro, lime juice, cumin, chili powder, salt, and pepper.
6. Cook for 5-7 minutes, or until heated through.
7. Cut sweet potatoes open and fill with the black bean mixture.
8. Serve immediately.

Snacks Meal Plan

Sweet Treats

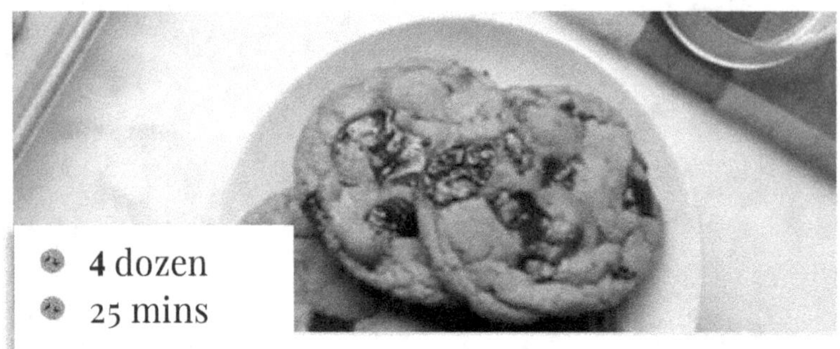

- **4** dozen
- **25** mins

Chocolate Chip Cookies

INGREDIENTS

1 cup (2 sticks) unsalted butter, softened

3/4 cup granulated sugar

3/4 cup packed light brown sugar

2 large eggs

1 teaspoon vanilla extract

2 1/4 cups all-purpose flour

1 teaspoon salt

1 teaspoon baking soda

1 cup semisweet chocolate chips

INSTRUCTIONS

1. Preheat oven to 375°F (190°C). Line baking sheets with parchment paper.
2. Cream butter and sugar in a large bowl until light and fluffy.
3. Beat in eggs one at a time, then add vanilla extract.
4. In a separate basin, mix flour, salt, and baking soda.
5. Gradually stir dry ingredients into wet ingredients until just mixed.
6. Stir in chocolate chips.
7. Drop tablespoons of dough onto prepared baking sheets, leaving about 2 inches between each cookie.
8. Bake for 10-12 minutes, or until golden brown around the edges.
9. Let cookies cool on baking sheets for a few minutes before transferring to a wire rack to cool completely.

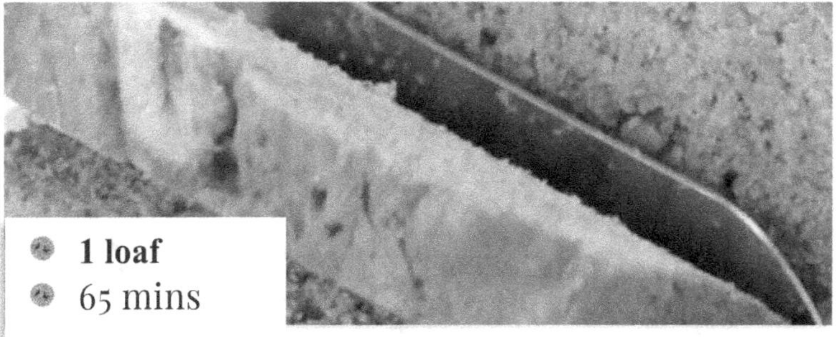

● **1 loaf**

● 65 mins

Peanut Butter Banana Bread

INGREDIENTS

1 1/2 cups all-purpose flour

1 teaspoon baking soda

1/2 teaspoon salt

1/2 cup unsalted butter, softened

1 cup granulated sugar

2 large eggs

1/2 cup mashed ripe bananas

1/3 cup creamy peanut butter

1/2 cup milk

INSTRUCTIONS

1. Preheat oven to 350°F (175°C). Grease and flour a 9x5 inch loaf pan.
2. whisk flour, baking soda, and salt together.
3. Cream butter and sugar in a large bowl until light and fluffy.
4. Beat in eggs one at a time, then stir in mashed bananas and peanut butter.
5. Alternately add dry ingredients and milk to wet ingredients, mixing until just combined.
6. Pour batter into prepared loaf pan.
7. Bake until a toothpick inserted into the center comes out clean or for 50-60 minutes.
8. Let bread cool in pan for 10 minutes before transferring to a wire rack to cool completely.

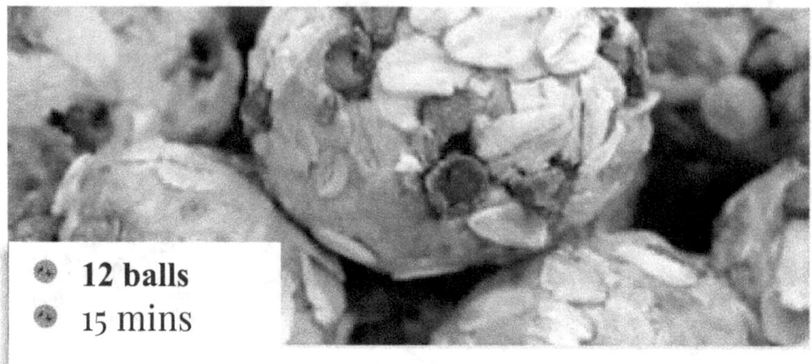

- **12 balls**
- 15 mins

No-Bake Energy Bites

INGREDIENTS

1 cup rolled oats
1/2 cup chopped nuts (e.g., almonds, pecans, walnuts)
1/4 cup unsweetened shredded coconut
1/4 cup dried fruit (e.g., raisins, cranberries, cherries)
1/4 cup honey
1/4 cup natural peanut butter
1 teaspoon vanilla extract

INSTRUCTIONS

1. In a large bowl, combine rolled oats, chopped nuts, shredded coconut, and dried fruit.
2. In a small saucepan, heat honey and peanut butter over low heat until melted and smooth.
3. Stir in vanilla extract.
4. Pour wet ingredients into dry ingredients and mix well until combined.
5. Roll mixture into balls.
6. Keep in an airtight container in the fridge for up to one week.

Savory Snacks

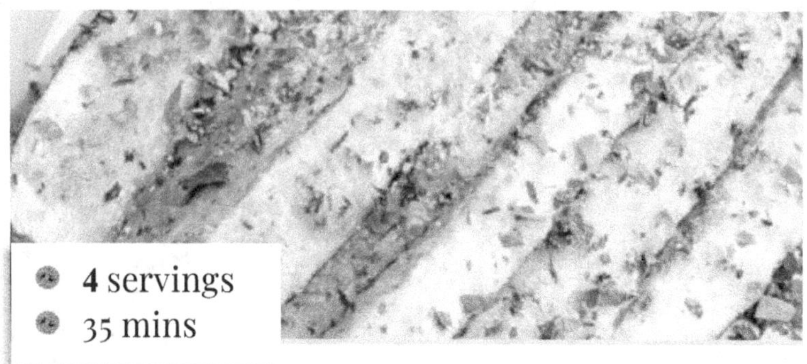

Baked Parmesan Zucchini Fries

INGREDIENTS

2 medium zucchinis, cut
into sticks

1/4 cup olive oil

1/4 cup grated Parmesan
cheese

1/4 teaspoon dried
oregano

1/4 teaspoon garlic
powder

1/4 teaspoon salt

1/4 teaspoon black pepper

INSTRUCTIONS

1. Preheat oven to 400°F (200°C). Prepare a baking sheet with parchment paper.
2. Toss zucchini sticks with olive oil, Parmesan cheese, oregano, garlic powder, salt, and pepper.
3. Spread zucchini sticks in a single layer on prepared baking sheet.
4. Bake for 20-25 minutes, or until golden brown and crispy.
5. Serve immediately.

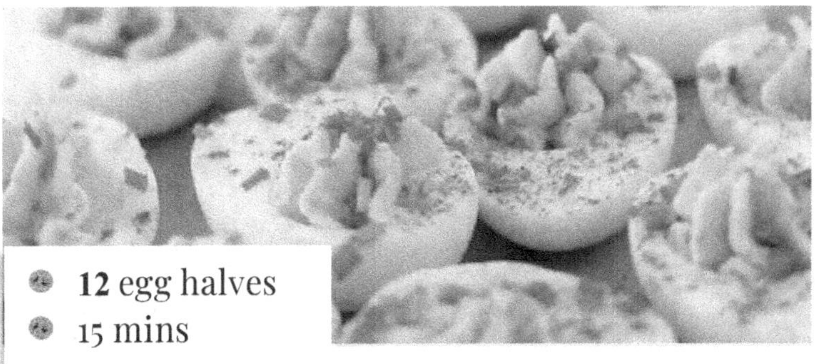

Smoked Paprika Deviled Eggs

INGREDIENTS

6 hard-boiled eggs, peeled and halved

1/4 cup mayonnaise

1 tablespoon Dijon mustard

1 teaspoon smoked paprika

1/4 teaspoon salt

1/4 teaspoon black pepper

Chopped fresh chives, for garnish (optional)

INSTRUCTIONS

1. Remove yolks from hard-boiled eggs and place in a bowl.
2. Mash yolks with a fork.
3. Stir in mayonnaise, Dijon mustard, smoked paprika, salt, and pepper.
4. Pipe or spoon the filling into the egg whites.
5. Garnish with chopped chives (optional).
6. Serve immediately or refrigerate for up to 24 hours

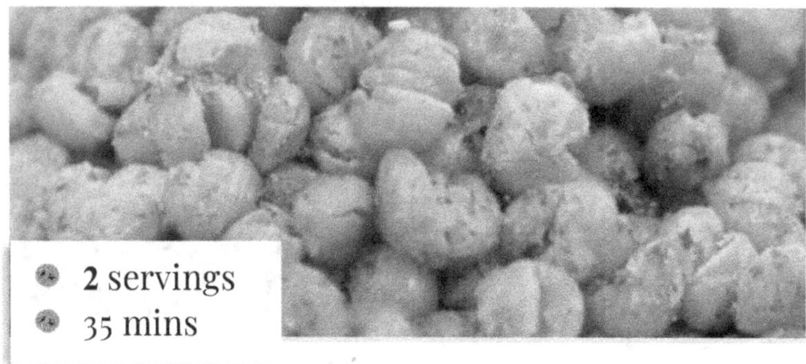

Spicy Roasted Chickpeas

INGREDIENTS

1 (15-ounce) can
chickpeas, drained and
rinsed

1 tablespoon olive oil

1 teaspoon chili powder

1/2 teaspoon smoked
paprika

1/4 teaspoon cayenne
pepper (optional)

1/4 teaspoon salt

1/4 teaspoon black pepper

INSTRUCTIONS

1. Preheat oven to 400°F (200°C). prepare a baking sheet with parchment paper.
2. Toss chickpeas with olive oil, chili powder, smoked paprika, cayenne pepper (if using), salt, and pepper.
3. Spread chickpeas in a single layer on prepared baking sheet.
4. Bake for 25-30 minutes, or until golden brown and crispy.
5. Serve immediately.

Healthy Dips & Spreads

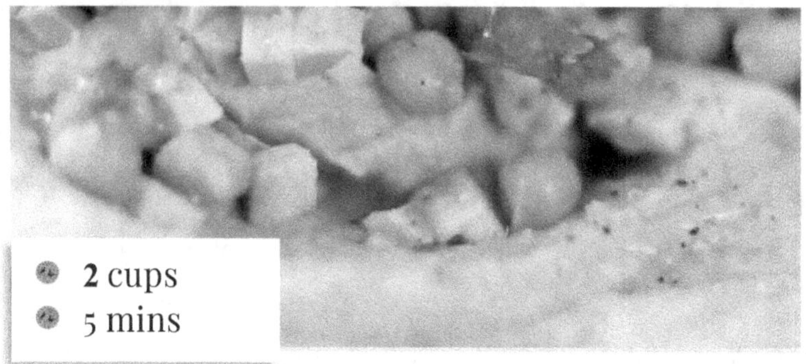

- **2** cups
- 5 mins

<u>Avocado Hummus</u>

INGREDIENTS

1 ripe avocado, pitted and peeled

1 (15-ounce) can chickpeas, drained and rinsed

1/4 cup tahini

1/4 cup olive oil

2 tablespoons lemon juice

1 clove garlic, minced

1/4 teaspoon salt

1/4 teaspoon black pepper

INSTRUCTIONS

1. Combine all ingredients in a blender or food processor.
2. Blend until smooth and creamy.
3. Serve with pita bread, vegetables, or crackers.

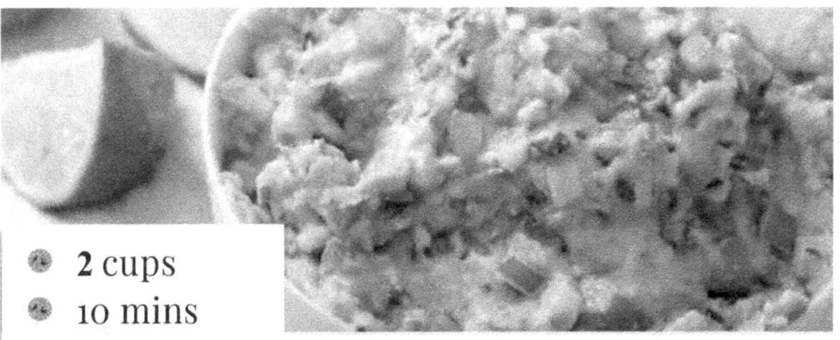

- **2** cups
- 10 mins

Homemade Guacamole

INGREDIENTS

2 ripe avocados, pitted and peeled

1/2 cup chopped red onion

1/4 cup chopped cilantro

2 tablespoons lime juice

1/2 teaspoon salt

1/4 teaspoon black pepper

INSTRUCTIONS

1. In a bowl, mash avocados using a fork.

2. Stir in red onion, cilantro, lime juice, salt, and pepper.

3. Serve with tortilla chips, vegetables, or crackers.

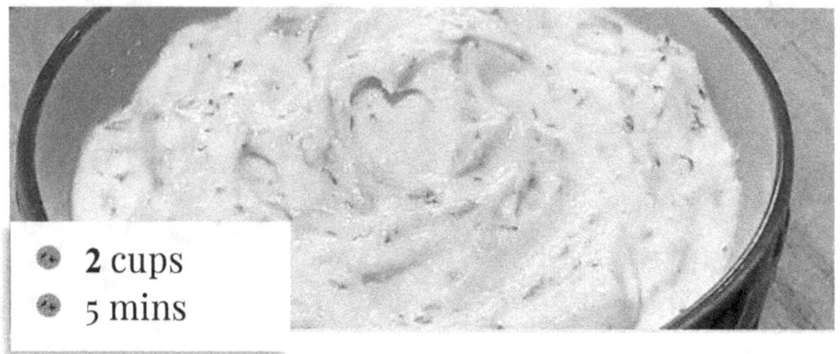

Greek Yogurt Ranch Dip

INGREDIENTS

1 cup plain Greek yogurt

1/4 cup mayonnaise

1 tablespoon chopped fresh dill

1 tablespoon chopped fresh chives

1 teaspoon dried onion powder

1 teaspoon garlic powder

1/2 teaspoon salt

1/4 teaspoon black pepper

INSTRUCTIONS

1. In a bowl, mix all ingredients and whisk until smooth.

2. Serve with vegetables, crackers, or pretzels.

CONCLUSION

You've embarked on a path not just towards leaner jeans and brighter mornings, but towards a vibrant, sustainable lifestyle. But the journey doesn't end here. Let's explore the steps to keep your low-carb, high-protein flame burning bright:

Maintaining the Momentum

Cravings are temporary, but your intuition deserves attention. opt for healthy swaps, find satiating low-carb alternatives, and prioritize sleep and hydration.

Experiment with new recipes, explore different cuisines, and keep your taste buds dancing. Your cookbook is your launchpad, not your limit!

Stock your pantry with low-carb staples, whip up batch meals for busy days, and pack satisfying snacks for on-the-go moments. Preparation paves the path to success.

Notice your clearer skin, boosted energy, improved sleep, and newfound confidence. These intangible victories are testaments to your transformation.

Sharing the Spark

Cook low-carb feasts for friends and family, share your favorite recipes, and become a beacon of healthy living. Your enthusiasm is contagious!

Join online communities and Connect with fellow low-carb enthusiasts, share tips and recipes, and offer support. Together, you can build a thriving community of cheerleaders.

You've equipped yourself with knowledge, satiated your taste buds with delicious recipes, and empowered yourself to thrive.

And as you recommend this cookbook to friends and family, whisper this promise: "It's not just a collection of recipes, it's a gateway to a healthier, happier you."

So, dear reader, go forth, conquer your health goals, and remember, we're all in this delicious, transformative journey together!

Appendix

Alphabetical index of all recipes.

A

B

C

D

G

T

V

30 DAYS MEAL PLAN

From   to

Monday

Friday

Tuesday

Saturday

Wednesday

Sunday

Thursday

Notes

30 Days Meal Plan

From   to

Monday	Friday
Tuesday	Saturday
Wednesday	Sunday
Thursday	Notes

30 Days Meal Plan

From   to

Monday	Friday
Tuesday	Saturday
Wednesday	Sunday
Thursday	Notes

30 Days Meal Plan

From   to

Monday

Friday

Tuesday

Saturday

Wednesday

Sunday

Thursday

Notes

Day 29

Day 30

www.ingramcontent.com/pod-product-compliance
Lightning Source LLC
Chambersburg PA
CBHW050737260726
48661CB00001B/281